Sleep with Buteyko

The only way to stop snoring,
sleep apnoea, and insomnia

Suitable for children,
teenagers and adults

PATRICK MCKEOWN
www.Snoring.ie

Published by: Buteyko Books
Loughwell, Moycullen, Co Galway, Ireland
Web: www.ButeykoClinic.com
Email: info@Buteykoclinic.com

© Patrick McKeown 2011

Cover design by Aurora Pérez Machío from www.apm-graphics.com

Illustrations by Rebecca Burgess from www.RebeccaBurgess.co.uk

ISBN-13: 9780956682376

Sleep that knits up the ravelled sleeve of care
The death of each day's life, sore labour's bath
Balm of hurt minds, great nature's second
course, Chief nourisher in life's feast.
~William Shakespeare, Macbeth

PROLOGUE

You are about to read a book containing complete
instructions on how to apply the Buteyko Method to stop
snoring, sleep apnoea, and insomnia. Bookstores are filled
with numerous self-help books on sleep-related disorders.
The vast majority, however, are missing a crucial link in
getting to the crux of the problem.

Unless chronic overbreathing is recognised and corrected,
one is scratching the surface and at most will only achieve
minor improvements. This book teaches you how to
reverse chronic hyperventilation, which plays a major role
in snoring, sleep apnoea, and insomnia, and will provide a
wealth of information needed to experience a better
night's sleep.

Numerous illustrations and a conversational style lighten
the message and add a visual impact. I hope that I have
created a snappy, easy-to-read, and well informed book.

All characters appearing in this work are fictitious.
Any resemblance to real persons, living or dead, is
purely coincidental.

CONTENTS

BOOK ONE

BOOK TWO

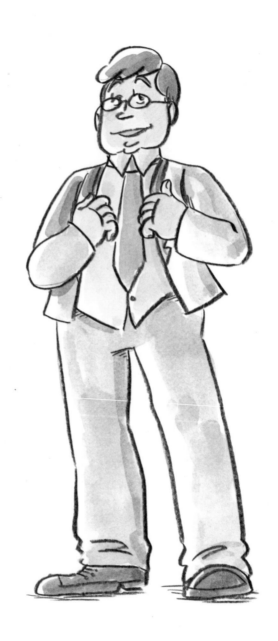

MEET CHIEF

Chief held a very respectable position on the island, as he was responsible for finance.

He enjoyed fine food and drink and did as little exercise as possible, and it showed. However, Chief was content and the populace held him in good esteem.

Over the years, his indulgent living began to show signs; he had put on more than just a few pounds, his face had rounded like a football, his belly was getting fat, and his neck was growing wide. But Chief was a likeable enough character, and was direct and to the point. And when the Chief slept at night, he snored. His snoring was so loud that he could be heard a number of rooms away. His snoring was like thunder.

Lately, not only did the Chief snore. He also grunted, gasped, and snorted during his sleep.

He snored loudly, which was then followed by complete silence. During the silence, his tummy and chest jerked and heaved as if attempting to draw air into his lungs. For many seconds, Chief did not breathe at all. His airways temporarily closed, and no air could enter or leave his body. Eventually, he resumed breathing with a large gasp of air.

The Chief's wife was growing concerned, as she heard this racket each night.

Like most people with severe snoring or sleep apnoea, Chief was completely oblivious to his condition. Each morning, he was sure that he was fine after a good night's sleep. He was beginning to notice, however, that he felt sluggish when he awoke. No longer was a mug of coffee enough to get him going. He was tired, had brain fog, and just didn't feel right.

As the months progressed, Chief often woke up with a headache, was more irritable than his usual self, and could sleep anywhere. Despite his responsibility for finance on the Island, the Chief slept when the returns came in. He slept when the island was falling into a crisis.
He slept when public spending continued. In fact, he spent most of his waking life falling asleep. Chief had the most important job on the island but was barely awake to do it. His disturbances during the night were preventing him from enjoying a deep, restful sleep.

Now, his interviews were in shambles. His words were sluggish and he sounded so nasally, as if he was talking through his nose. During one morning interview, he sounded so bad that it became the talk of the island. The Island Times newspaper reported that Chief was exhausted.

Chief had enough. The island was now in crisis and he simply had to improve his energy level. Being sleepy was OK when everything was rosy. When citizens were spending plenty, Chief could put his feet up.

Now, however, spending had stopped. Banks had no money. Builders could not sell their houses. Auctioneers were closing their shops. Thousands of people were out of work.

It was time for Chief to WAKE UP.

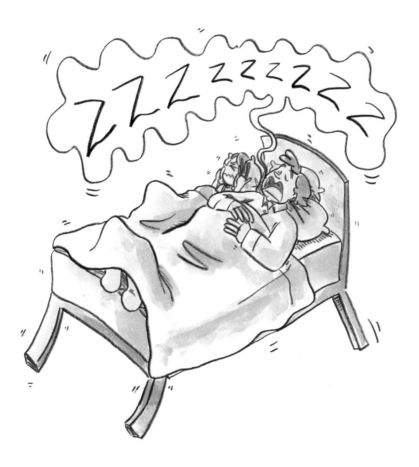

MEET BUTEYKO

The Buteyko Method was developed in the 1950s by Russian doctor Konstantin Buteyko. Hundreds of thousands of people have practised his method for a variety of conditions including asthma, high blood pressure, sleeping difficulties, anxiety, stress, panic attacks and depression.

As a young doctor, Buteyko spent many months sitting at sick patients' bedsides, observing their states of health. He noticed that each person's breathing got heavier as his or her health deteriorated. As their illnesses advanced, he saw that his patients' breathing movements from their chests and tummies increased, that their breathing became more audible, that their breaths became faster and that they sighed more and breathed more frequently through their mouths.

This raised a fundamental question for Buteyko: did his patients' sickness contribute to their heavy breathing or did their heavy breathing contribute to their sickness?

At the time, Buteyko suffered from severe hypertension that continued to worsen. He began experimenting by breathing less and quietening his breathing. Within a short while, the pains that he had experienced for months disappeared.

Over the following decades, Buteyko extensively researched this subject and operated a dedicated laboratory to further his findings. His method was brought to the West in 1990 and is now taught in many countries.
Breathing, such a vital factor for life, must meet certain conditions. Severe overbreathing can be fatal if sustained over a short period. Therefore, it is plausible to accept that negative health effects result from less severe but still excessive breathing over a long period.

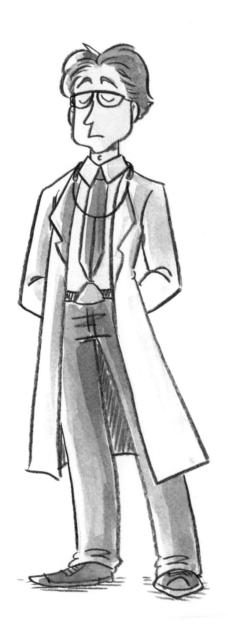

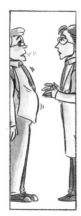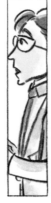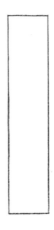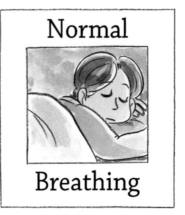

Normal

Breathing

Before Buteyko guides Chief through his method,
let's briefly look at what normal breathing is,
and describe snoring, sleep apnoea and insomnia.

WHAT IS NORMAL BREATHING?

Did you know that the number of breaths per minute during normal breathing is about 10 to 12?

Each breath takes in approximately 500 ml of air. As described in any university medical textbook, this amount provides a healthy volume of five to six litters of air per minute. A normal breathing pattern is quiet, still, calm, relaxed, and regular.

People suffering from snoring and sleep apnoea breathe in more air than the normally accepted amounts. For example, this group commonly takes 15 to 20 breaths per minute, with each breath taking in more than the normal 500 ml of air. Assuming that each breath is 700 ml, the average breathing volume for this person is 10 to 15 litres of air per minute. In food terms, this is akin to eating six to nine meals each day!

This over-breathing or hyper-ventilation does not add any more oxygen to the blood, as it is normally 97–98% saturated. Instead, it causes a loss of the gas carbon dioxide. Carbon dioxide is not just a waste gas. For oxygen to be released from the red blood cells, carbon dioxide must be present. Suffice to say that the heavier you breathe, the less oxygen is delivered to tissues and organs.

Listen to the breathing of someone who snores or has sleep apnoea. Without a doubt, you will find it to be heavy, noisy and loud.

WHAT CAUSES SNORING?

Snoring, often the subject of jokes about rattling the windows and waking the baby, has a much more serious side. Left untreated, snoring may progress into sleep apnoea, high blood pressure or cardiovascular complaints. Not to mention the disruption it causes to sleeping partners.

Simply, snoring is a sound created from turbulent airflow. It is noisy breathing during sleep caused by the exchange of a large volume of air through a narrowed space, which in turn causes the tissues of the nose and throat to vibrate. Snoring can affect any member of the family, regardless of age, from granny to toddler. An estimated 45% of men and 30% of women snore habitually.

The question to ask is whether you would snore if your breathing was calm and quiet?

Healthy non-snorers breathe quietly through their nose. Their sleep is deep and undisturbed, and they wake up refreshed.

People who breathe heavily during the night experience a wide array of symptoms, such as snoring, sleep apnoea, disrupted sleep, insomnia, needing to use the toilet, and waking up fatigued with a dry mouth and a possible blocked nose.

Snorers snore through their mouth, their nose, or both their nose and mouth.

Snoring through the mouth is the easiest to address. Such

snoring stops when one learns to breathe through his or her nose during sleep.

Snoring through the nose stops when one unblocks the nose and corrects his or her breathing volume to normal levels. By learning to unblock the nose, switching to nasal breathing, and normalising breathing volume, breathing will be quiet, calm, and still throughout the night and nasal snoring will cease.

While most treatments for snoring such as nasal decongestants, nasal strips, surgery and dental appliances aim to expand the airways to make more room for airflow, this book in addition to expanding the airways normalises breathing volume.

THE WORLD'S LOUDEST SNORER

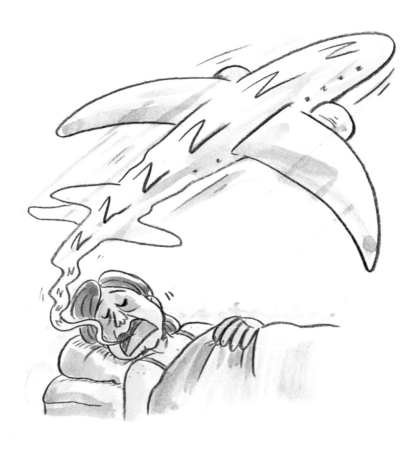

The British newspaper, The Telegraph, reported the following.

"Mrs Chapman, 60, snores every night at 111.6 decibels - eight decibels louder than the roar of a low-flying jet - much to the dismay of long suffering husband Colin, 62.

The retired bank worker could drown out the sounds of a spinning washing machine, diesel truck, farm tractor or speeding express train.

She regularly wakes herself up and her husband Colin has had to retreat to the spare room at least five nights a week for the 18 years they have been married.

She has snored throughout her entire life and one of her earliest memories is waking up to her sister pinching the bridge of her nose when she was five.

Over the years Mrs Chapman has tried nose bands, pills, visited the doctor "countless" times and even considered invasive surgery in a bid to cure her snoring." [1]

If you know Mrs Chapman, please give her a copy of this book.

SNORING IN THE WILD WEST

Snoring is more than just a minor inconvenience. During the 1800's in the American Wild West, there was once a notorious gunfighter named John Wesley Hardin.

Hardin was asleep one night at the American House Hotel. In the adjoining room, a man snored so loudly that it kept Hardin awake.

In a fit of rage, Hardin fired several bullets through the wall and ceiling of the bedroom. It is said that the first bullet merely woke the man; the second killed him.

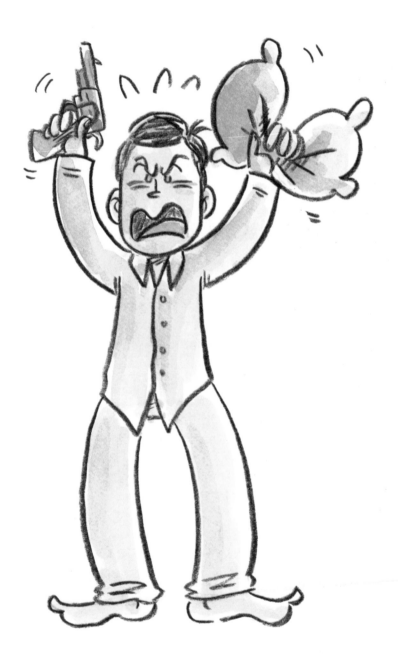

WHAT CAUSES SLEEP APNOEA?

A pnoea is a Greek word meaning "without breath."

There are three types of apnoea during sleep: central, obstructive and mixed.
Mixed apnoea is a combination of central and obstructive sleep apnoea. It can be argued with some conviction that chronic hyperventilation offers an explanation for both types of sleep apnoea.

Central Sleep Apnoea
Central sleep apnoea affects approximately 5% of sufferers and results from the brain not sending the right signals to breathe. Excessive breathing volume during sleep causes a reduction in the partial pressure of carbon dioxide. This shifts the pH of the blood in an alkaline direction. To maintain the pH within normal levels, a natural bodily response is to hold the breath, allowing the pH to revert to normal. In other words, central apnoea occurs from breathing in excess of metabolic requirements.

Obstructive Sleep Apnoea
During your school days, you may remember reading about Joe the "fat boy" from the Pickwick papers written by Charles Dickens in 1837.

Joe ate in great quantities and was liable to fall asleep during any situation. His breathing was heavy, he snored and he was continuously sleepy. Originally described as the Pickwickian syndrome, his breathing was later labelled as obstructive sleep apnoea syndrome.

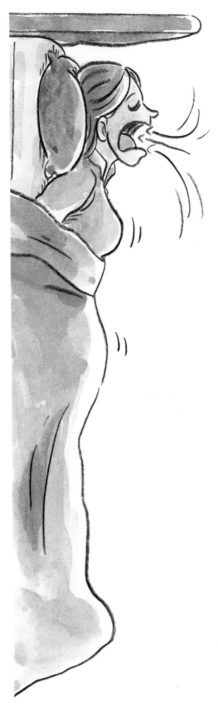

While obstructive sleep apnoea more often affects men with a neck size of 17 inches or larger, it can also affect children and adults who are not overweight.

Children who breathe through their mouth are at risk of developing cranio-facial changes, such as undeveloped jaws, smaller airways, and narrow faces. This increases the likelihood of the child developing lifelong sleep apnoea.

Obstructive sleep apnoea is the most common type of apnoea and is characterised by holding the breath from collapse of the upper airways during sleep. This holding of the breath, which prevents airflow to the lungs, may occur between five and fifty times per hour. Each breath hold can range from a few seconds to over one minute, causing one's blood oxygen saturation to decline to as low as 50%.

After a period of holding the breath during sleep, the centre within the brain that controls breathing alerts the rest of the brain that the breath is being held and the individual partially wakes up. This is followed by gasping, a sharp intake of breath, and spluttering, which is often of great concern to sleep partners who in turn suffer from sleep deprivation. The sufferer is unaware that he or she is holding his or her breath, often feels that he or she slept well but wonders why he or she is so tired during the day.

All patients with sleep apnoea breathe extremely heavily while sleeping. A normal routine is thunderous snoring followed by complete cessation of the breath.

Imagine sucking air through a collapsible rubber tube. As one sucks air through the tube, the walls of the tube tend to collapse inwards from the pressure created by drawing air. During a gentle draw of air, pressure is minimal and the inner walls of the tube do not collapse. However, during a strong draw of air, the walls can collapse and the more effort one makes to suck air through the tube, the more the walls collapse.

An engineer looking at this problem might offer two solutions. The first is to widen the tube. The second is to reduce the airflow.

Widening a human airway through surgery is a last resort. While losing weight from around the neck region is helpful, a more plausible option is to reduce breathing volume.

Mouth and excessive breathing causes the airway walls to collapse, resulting in holding of the breath. During the cessation of the breath, the chest and diaphragm continue to try to draw air into the lungs. This results in jerking and heaving as the diaphragm presses downward. The greater the heaving of the chest and diaphragm, the more the airway walls are drawn inward. Eventually, the patient begins to breathe again.

Symptoms resulting from sleep apnoea include excessive daytime sleepiness, waking up tired, loud snoring, holding the breath during the night, loud snorts, gasps upon resumption of breathing, dry throat, dry mouth, and headaches in morning, problems with memory and concentration, heartburn or reflux, swelling of the legs, needing to urinate during the night, sweating during sleep, chest pain, and elevations in blood pressure. Of course, this loud snoring accompanied by loud snorts and gasps can also lead to marital problems.

WHAT IS INSOMNIA?

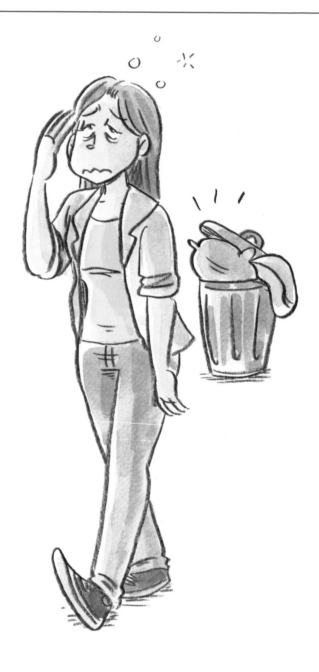

Chronic overbreathing disturbs blood gases resulting in excessive brain cell excitability leading to random and excessive thoughts. This in turn contributes to insomnia.

Insomnia is a state where you are never fully asleep and never fully awake.

People with insomnia may find it difficult to fall asleep, may wake up a number of times during the night, may wake up too early in the morning, and may feel very tired upon waking. Disrupted sleep results in daytime fatigue and can lead to anxiety and depression.

Symptoms of insomnia include slowing down, daytime moodiness, sleepiness during the day, general tiredness, irritability, and problems with concentration or memory.

It is estimated that one in ten adults suffer from insomnia and this increases to one in five adults over the age of 65.

In the next section of the book, Buteyko meets Chief and guides him through the effects of overbreathing, how to recognise it and how to reverse it. To create a more userfriendly experience, part of the text is written in conversation style.

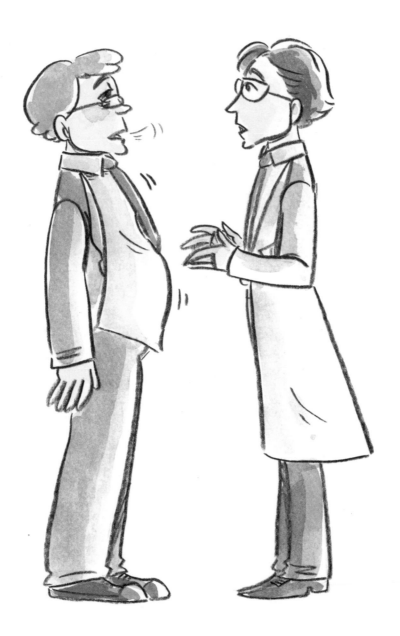

CHIEF IS CHRONICALLY OVERBREATHING!

Buteyko explained to Chief: "Quite simply, your lifestyle over the years has changed your breathing. Now you breathe through your mouth day and night. You sigh and snort regularly, and take large breaths prior to talking. Your breathing is noisy, and I can see visible movements in your tummy and chest when you breathe."

"And, of course, when you breathe heavily during the day, you will breathe heavily at night. Chief, you are here to address your snoring, sleep apnoea and insomnia. Surprisingly, they are all related to each other, and have a single causal factor, namely overbreathing!"

Buteyko used very simple terminology to get his point across.

"Now, Chief, if you drink too much, what happens?"

Chief replied: "I get drunk."

"Yes, you get drunk. And if you eat too much, what happens?"

Chief: "I feel sick and sluggish."

"Yes, that is right. And I am going to tell you something else: your over drinking, overeating, lack of exercise, stress, stuffy rooms and excessive talking is making you overbreathe. And your overbreathing is severely affecting your health. It causes your nose to become blocked and your blood vessels and airways to constrict, it disrupts your sleep and it results in snoring, sleep apnoea and insomnia."

OVERBREATHING CAUSES POOR CONCENTRATION

Buteyko continued: "Is it true that your concentration is not nearly as good as it used to be? Concentration is our ability to focus all of our attention on the task at hand without internal distractions. For example, if we are reading a report, we can follow the report without random thoughts interrupting us. That is why this book is very visual, to assist with poor concentration originating from sleep disturbances."

"DO YOU FIND THAT YOUR CONCENTRATION IS GOOD?"

Chief replied: "No, it is not nearly as good as it used to be. Ever since my snoring worsened and I began to gasp and grunt during my sleep, my concentration has changed. My mind wanders a lot. When faced with an unknown situation, I am unable to solve it whereas before I could. It seems that my entire brain has slowed down."

"Buteyko, you are telling me that heavy breathing is bad for me, that it causes my airways to close, my snoring and my insomnia. And this results in my sleepiness, poor concentration, headaches and bad mood. But everybody I meet talks about taking a deep breath and filling my lungs with oxygen. How can I be sure that what you are telling me is true?"

Buteyko explained that none of these people understand how oxygen is released from red blood cells. "If they knew about the Bohr effect, they wouldn't advocate heavy breathing or taking big breaths."

Buteyko continued: "When Lavoisier discovered oxygen, he likened the human body to fire. Just like fire, the human organism consumes oxygen and gives off carbon dioxide. However, this is not the complete story. Not all oxygen is good, which is why we have antioxidants. Not all carbon dioxide is bad, as normal bodily functions are very dependent on this gas. It is very important that we have the correct partial pressure of both within our body. However, when we breathe in excess of bodily requirements, our health is negatively affected"

Buteyko told Chief to forget about the theory and asks him how he feels when he breathes heavily through his mouth for a few minutes.

Chief knows only too well. "When I do that, I feel dizzy and light headed. My brain does not function as well. I also find that I have a slight pain in my heart region."
Buteyko is happy that Chief has discovered the connection between his heavy breathing and health.

Most people in the Western world overbreathe. It is a factor of modern living, but how it affects each individual depends on genetic predisposition.

Buteyko asked Chief whether he wakes up tired in the morning. Chief replied:
"Yes, I do."

Buteyko explained that this is related to the way he breathes. Breathing too much reduces oxygenation of the brain!

MAN AND HIS USELESS IDEAS ABOUT BREATHING!

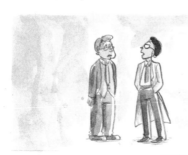

Chief, tell me this; if you go to the seaside for a walk with your dog,

does your dog increase his breathing because he believes that inhaling salty air is good for him?

No, my dog just breathes as he always does.

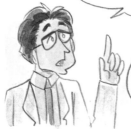

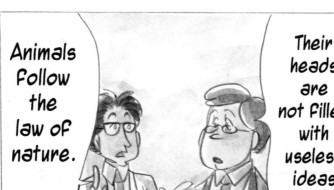

Animals follow the law of nature.

Their heads are not filled with useless ideas.

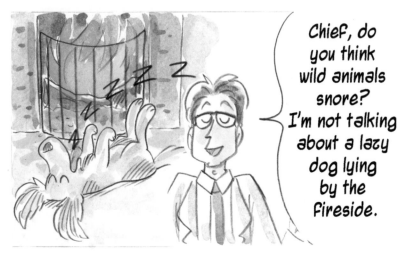

Chief, do you think wild animals snore? I'm not talking about a lazy dog lying by the fireside.

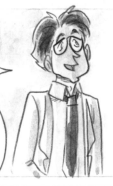

I am talking about an animal living in its natural environment.

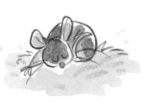

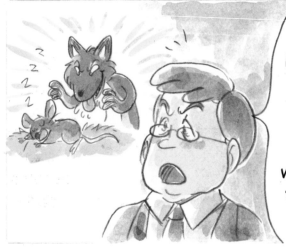

I don't imagine that an animal would. If it did, it would be very vulnerable to predators.

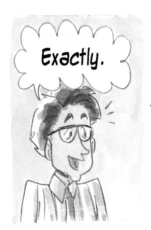

Exactly.

I hear that your daughter had a beautiful little baby girl two months ago.

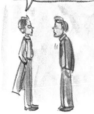

Does the baby breathe through her nose or mouth?

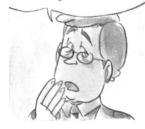

The baby breathes through its nose.

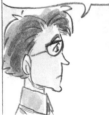

And can you hear the baby breathe?

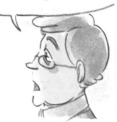

No, the baby's breathing is silent.

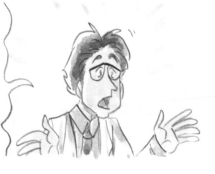

If your granddaughter was snoring thunderously, heaving, grunting and gasping during her sleep, would you be concerned?

Yes, very much so. That wouldn't seem a natural thing to do.

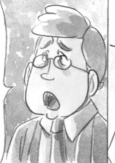

Would you say that such a baby is unhealthy?

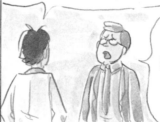

Yes.

Well, the same is true for adults. Why should an adult be different from a healthy baby?

I want you to breathe just like a healthy baby breathes.

I want you to breathe only through your nose.

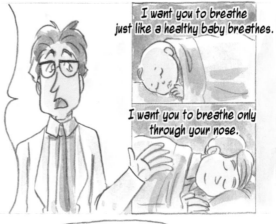

This is how you were breathing when you were born. I want you to watch your breathing and breathe quietly during the day.

But Buteyko,

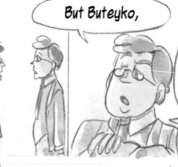

I find it difficult to believe that the answer to my problems is simply changing my breathing.

Surely, you are going to give me medication or perform surgery?

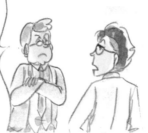

No, Chief. I am going to give you the tools to help you deal with your own health problems.

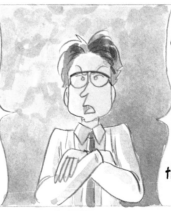

Surgery is a last resort for snoring and sleep apnoea, and often makes no difference whatsoever.

Websites sell every gimmick possible to address snoring but none of them produce the results that this will produce for you.

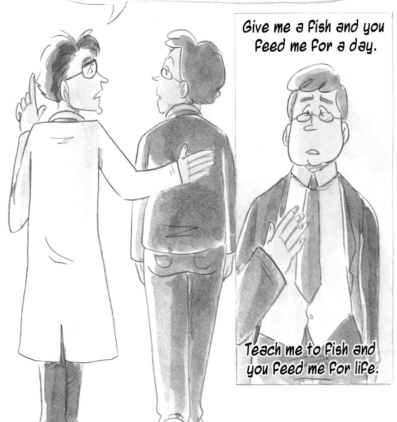

It is high time that you took responsibility for your own health. There is an old Chinese proverb:

Give me a fish and you feed me for a day.

Teach me to fish and you feed me for life.

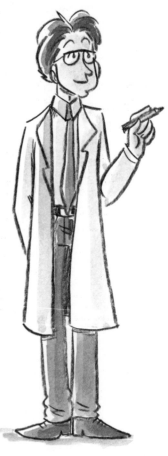

Good breathing is quiet.

Good breathing is calm.

Good breathing is invisible.

Good breathing is in and out through our nose.

Not good breathing is through the mouth.

Not good breathing is sighing, snorting, and sniffing while resting.

Not good breathing is visible movements of the chest and tummy.

Not good breathing is noisy breathing.

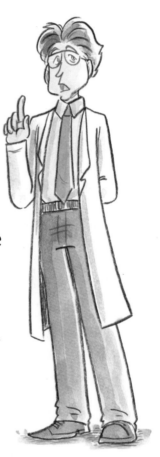

HOW TO MEASURE YOUR RELATIVE BREATHING VOLUME

Buteyko explained to Chief that a measurement called the control pause (CP) was developed to measure relative breathing volume. Quite simply, it is the length of comfortable breath hold time following an exhalation. All you need is a watch or clock with a second hand.

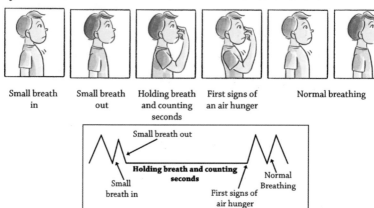

Small breath in	Small breath out	Holding breath and counting seconds	First signs of an air hunger	Normal breathing

1. Take a small, silent breath in and a small, silent breath out.
2. Hold your nose with your fingers to prevent air from entering your lungs.
3. Count how many seconds until you feel the first signs of air hunger.
4. At the first sign of air hunger, you will also feel the first involuntary movements of your breathing muscles. Your tummy may jerk.
   The area around your neck may contract.
5. Release your nose and breathe in through it.
6. Your inhalation at the end of the breath should be calm.

The following are important points to be aware of before we start:

1.   The breath is taken after gently exhaling.
2.   The breath is held until the first movements of the breathing muscles. It is not a measure of the maximum length of time that you can hold your breath.
3.   Your CP only measures your breath hold time. It is not an exercise to correct your breathing.

Remember that taking your CP entails holding your breath only until the first involuntary movements of your breathing muscles. If you had to take a big breath at the end of the breath hold, then you held your breath for too long.

THE THREE STEPS TO INCREASING YOUR CONTROL PAUSE

STEP 1
Stop Big Breathing

a. Breathe through your nose permanently

b. Stop Sighing – swallow or suppress the sigh

c. Never hear your breathing during rest

STEP 2
Practice reduced breathing (explained further on)

STEP 3
Take physical exercise with correct breathing (explained further on)

In summary;

To increase your CP from 10 - 20 seconds, STEPS 1 and 2 are necessary.

To increase your CP from 20 – 40 seconds, STEP 3 is necessary.

The following are essential rules to making progress.

- You will feel better each time your CP increases by five seconds.

- If your CP does not change, you will not feel better.

- Your CP should increase by three to four seconds each week.

- The most accurate CP is taken first thing after waking. This CP is most accurate since you cannot influence your breathing during sleep, and it is based on your breathing volume as set by your respiratory centre.

- Taking your CP throughout the day will give you feedback at those particular times.

- Your goal is to have a morning CP of 40 seconds for six months.

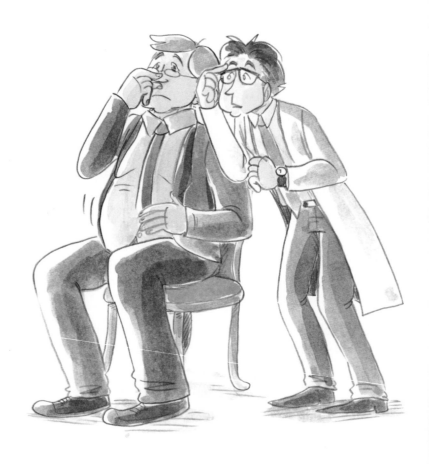

Chief measured his control pause, while Buteyko monitored whether he did it correctly by observing the first movements or contractions of his neck. Chief let go of his nose at the first movements of his breathing muscles. His control pause was 13 seconds.

Buteyko explained: "Chief, your control pause is 13 seconds which means that you are breathing for about four people." Chief was amazed, so Buteyko explained that he got this figure by dividing the control pause number into sixty.

For example, a control pause of ten seconds indicates that one is breathing a volume of air for six people while a control pause of twenty seconds indicates a breathing volume for three people.

Buteyko continued to explain that the ideal control pause is sixty seconds, while a control pause between 40 and 60 seconds is good.

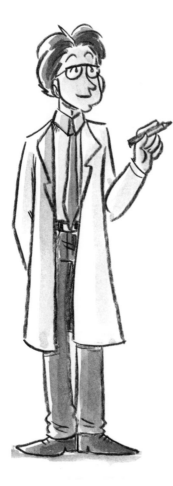

The three tenets to normalising your breathing:

1. Close your mouth and breathe through your nose day and night.

2. Adopt the correct posture.

3. Relax the inner body, the chest, and the tummy to create an ar shortage.

THE FIRST TENET: BREATHE THROUGH YOUR NOSE DAY AND NIGHT

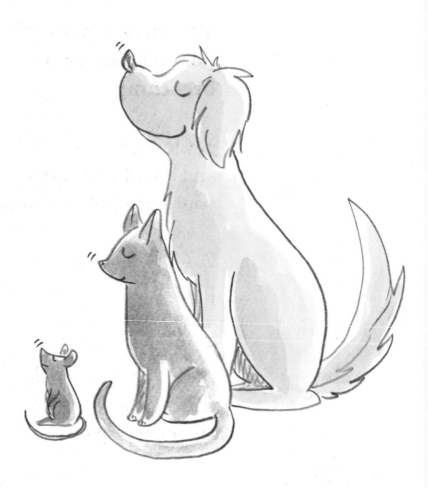

L earning to breathe permanently through the nose is the first step to addressing overbreathing. The nose serves a number of very important functions, including the following;

- It warms and humidifies incoming air.
- It removes a significant amount of germs and bacteria.
- It results in more regular breathing (chaotic breathing disturbs blood gases, which can play a role in experiencing stress).
- Breathing through the mouth results in a dry mouth, which increases acidification of the mouth and results in more dental cavities and gum disease.
- Breathing through the mouth causes dehydration.
- Breathing through the mouth has been proven to significantly increase the number of occurrences of and severity of apnoeas. (more in Book two)
- Breathing through the mouth is a significant cause of snoring.

In addition, children who breathe through their mouth develop lifelong craniofacial changes. When the mouth is closed, the resting position of the tongue is at the roof of the mouth. Each time you swallow, the tongue moves upwards and is flattened in the roof of the mouth; the action that forms the shape of the top jaw.
A well-developed top jaw is U-shaped, and optimally houses all teeth.

Conversely, when the mouth is open, the tongue rests midway or on the floor of the mouth. The top jaw does not receive the stimulation from the tongue, causing it to become narrow and V-shaped. A narrow, undeveloped V-shaped top jaw increases the risk of the child developing lifelong sleep apnoea.

The book entitled *Buteyko Meets Dr. Mew* brings together the life's work of renowned orthodontist Dr. Mew and explores this topic in great detail.

While it is very important that the mouth is closed during the day, it is absolutely vital that the mouth is closed during sleep. A closed mouth during sleep helps ensure that the tongue rests at the roof of the mouth. Conversely, when we sleep with our mouth open, the tongue falls back and makes the airway smaller, causing the floppy bits to vibrate loudly with each inhalation, which results in snoring. When the sagging of the oropharynx develops into a total inward collapse of the airways, the sleeper becomes unable to breathe and has an apnoea.

It is well documented that nasal obstruction and breathing through the mouth are significant causal factors for snoring and sleep apnoea. The science can be found in book two.

HOW TO UNBLOCK YOUR NOSE

Buteyko: Chief, I have to say that during every interview you have, I can sense that your nose is blocked.

Chief: Yes, that is why I breathe through my mouth.

Buteyko: Well, I will show you how to free it. The only reason your nose is blocked is because you are breathing too much. The more you breathe through your mouth, the more that your nose will be blocked. When you breathe too much, the partial pressure of carbon dioxide in your lungs and blood reduces. This causes a pooling of blood in the nose, increases swelling and creates more mucus.

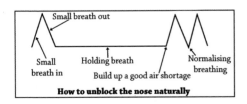

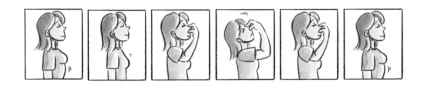

How to unblock the nose naturally

Buteyko: So, to unblock your nose, do the opposite of big breathing. Hold your breath on the out breath instead. Here is how to do this.

- Take a small breath in through your nose.

- Allow a small breath out through your nose.

- Hold your nose with your fingers to prevent air from entering or escaping.

- Nod your head up and down or sway your body until you feel a very strong need for air.

- Hold your breath for as long as you comfortably can.

- Let go and breathe in through your nose.

- Calm your breath immediately.

Wait for one minute and repeat. Repeat five or six times until your nose is completely free. And at any time that your nose gets blocked, repeat this again to temporarily decongest your nose. Your nose will be permanently free when you experience a high control pause.

NASAL BREATHE DURING SLEEP

Chief: "Yes, Buteyko, I will begin to keep my mouth closed. But what will I do at night? How can I keep my mouth closed at night while I sleep?"
"I will give you this paper tape. It is one-inch paper tape that you can buy at any chemist. The brand that I like is 3M Micropore. If you are not sure of how to apply the tape, I have a free video that shows you how, you can watch it at ButeykoDVD.com.

This is how you put it on. Tear off about six inches or ten centimetres. Fold over a small piece at one end of the tape to make removing it easier. Dry your lips with your hand. Draw your lips inwards and place the tape horizontally to cover your mouth. Go to sleep with your mouth closed."

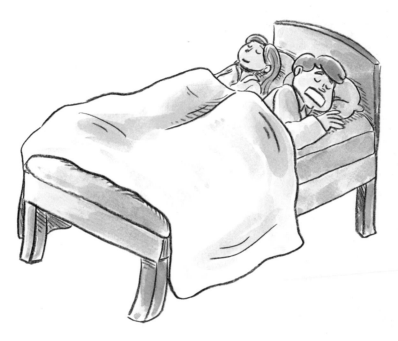

Chief: "Buteyko, I tried taping my mouth last night but I felt like I wasn't getting enough air."

Buteyko: "Well, there is a simple answer to that. You are feeling like you not getting enough air because you have been breathing so heavily through your mouth for the past fifty years. Your body has gotten used to your heavy breathing. But you will need only a very short time before you get used to breathing through your nose."

"Because you are feeling suffocated while breathing through your nose during sleep, I want you to wear a plastic strip to dilate your nose. This is only temporary and will make the transition a little easier. One brand is called breathe right strips, but you can find similar brands at your local chemist."

"Wear the paper tape across your mouth and the strip across your nose. This may not help your romantic life, but it will certainly help your sleep. After a couple of weeks, when your breathing becomes quieter, you won't need to wear the plastic strip as your nose will be naturally dilated and your breathing volume will have gone down."

THE SECOND TENET: CORRECT POSTURE

Buteyko explained that the second tenet is to display good posture. "Slouching over compresses our diaphragm and breathing moves more to the upper chest. This activates the sympathetic nervous system, resulting in greater stress and increased breathing volume. Be aware of your posture when you sit."

"The ideal sitting position is horse rider, where you sit at the edge of chair with your feet tucked under the chair. Imagine a thread drawing you upwards from the top of the back of your head. Imagine the spaces between your ribs widening. Be aware of your posture when you sit, walk, and run."

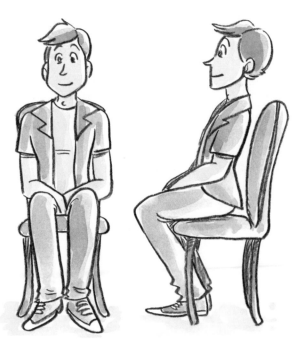

THE THIRD TENET: CREATE NEED FOR AIR

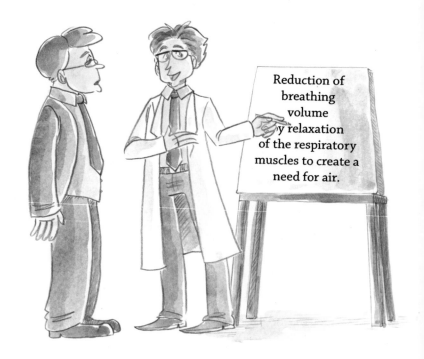

Reduction of breathing volume y relaxation of the respiratory muscles to create a need for air.

B uteyko explained the third tenet to Chief, which is to create a need for air through relaxation of the respiratory muscles.

To normalise your breathing volume, you need to practise special exercises to relax your body. This is done by bringing relaxation to your body and silently encouraging your breathing to decrease to the point where you feel a hunger for air. With a sustained shortage of air, the breathing centre is reset to direct more calm and gentle breathing. The more you keep your breathing quiet, the more this becomes your permanent way to breathe.

Chief: "Buteyko, I am confused; what is a hunger for air and how much should it be?"

Buteyko: "Hunger for air is wanting or needing air. It is a feeling of breathlessness, similar to what you would experience if you go for a walk. It can also be described as feeling slightly suffocated."

"Ideally, you have a tolerable need for air. The need for air should be the same as what you experience during your control pause. If you reduce your breathing too much, the air shortage is no longer tolerable and your breathing muscles jerk and heave. When the breathing muscles jerk, it is better for you to distract yourself for about thirty seconds and then resume gentle, reduced breathing through relaxation."

"Initially, you will be able to tolerate a shortage of air for a short period, maybe fifteen seconds or so, until the tummy jerks. However, with practise and as your control pause increases, it is far easier to maintain a gentle air shortage over a number of minutes."

Chief: "Okay, I will try it for a few minutes."

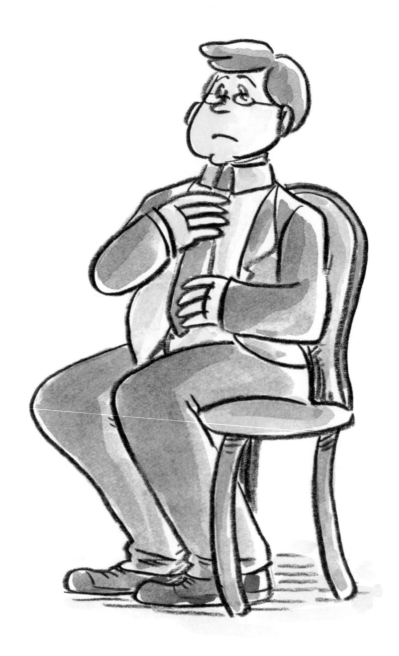

Chief put his hand on his chest and tummy and felt his breathing. He felt the air entering and leaving his nose. He felt the air hitting the back of the throat. He also felt his chest and tummy moving. To improve his awareness, Chief spent a number of minutes feeling the slightly cooler air entering his nose and the slightly warmer air leaving his nose.

When he had a good awareness of his breathing, Chief started to silently tell himself to "relax my chest," and "relax my tummy," for his "breathing to reduce," to "slow down," and "to quiet."

In addition to mental encouragement to relax, Chief brought inner relaxation to the area around his chest and tummy.

By relaxing, Chief took a smaller breath in than what he was used to and allowed a slow, gentle relaxed breath out. He felt his chest and tummy relaxing.

Small breath in, relaxed breath out
Small breath in, relaxed breath out
Small breath in, relaxed breath out

He mentally instructed his body to relax and, as his body relaxed, his breathing went quiet and calm.

Chief now had far less breathing movement from his neck downwards. His breathing was almost invisible but not quite. He felt a tolerable need or want for air.

Buteyko: "Chief, you are doing wonderfully well. You have a hunger for air. I know this because I can see that you are concentrating on your breathing. Your breathing movements have relaxed and have been reduced by about thirty per cent. I also know that you have air shortage because your eyes are glassy. There is a shine to them. Your face is pink, as the reduced breathing helps open up blood vessels and improves blood circulation. Finally, you have increased saliva in your mouth and I know this because you are swallowing more frequently."

SUMMARY

- Follow and feel your breathing for a minute or so

- Encourage the area around your chest and tummy to relax

- Bring relaxation to your inner body

- Silently encourage your breathing to slow down and go quiet

- Allow your breathing to reduce to the point that you feel a tolerable need for air

- Try to sustain this feeling for a few minutes

REDUCE BREATHING ONLY THROUGH RELAXATION OF THE RESPIRATORY MUSCLES

Chief was delighted that he was doing it correctly. He was so happy that he wanted to do more. He began to reduce his breathing further by deliberately tensing his tummy muscles. He tensed his muscles in his tummy to reduce his breathing. He also put the brakes to his breathing. This created a far stronger air shortage. Now his tummy started to jerk and his breathing rhythm was very disrupted.

Buteyko: "Chief you are doing it a little crudely at the moment. The real way to reduce your breathing is not through deliberate efforts at constricting your breathing movements by tensing the tummy or chest muscles. Breathing is not something that can be forced into place."

"By encouraging your body, chest, and tummy to relax, breathing automatically goes quieter. This alone can create a need for air. If it does not, then encourage your breathing to become quieter and more still. Encourage your breathing to slow down and relax. Encourage your breathing to reduce though mental commands and through inner relaxation. But don't tense your breathing muscles to create the need for air."

Chief: "Okay, Buteyko, I will do that."

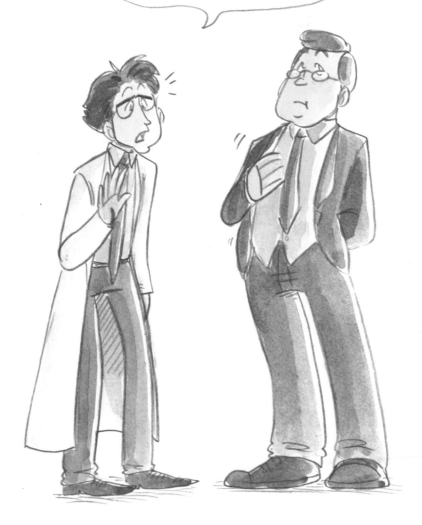

Buteyko: "Addressing chronic overbreathing not only stops snoring and sleep apnoea. It is also a wonderful way to eliminate insomnia; another very common sleep-related disorder. Insomnia simply means that you find it very difficult to fall asleep. For example, your mind may be thinking too much while you lie down at night and you may need an hour or two before you drop off."

"Another indication of insomnia is when you are awake during the night. You might wake up at 3 a.m. and feel that you are unable to get back to sleep."

"Later, I explain how overbreathing causes a disturbance of blood gases, resulting in increased nerve cell excitability, and random and excessive thoughts."

REDUCED BREATHING FORMAT

"Chief, I would like you to reduce your breathing for one formal session each day. A typical format for such a day is as follows:"

- Sit for five to ten minutes relaxing
- Measure your CP
- Practise five minutes of relaxation to create air shortage
- CP + 5 seconds
- Practise five minutes of relaxation to create air shortage
- CP + 10 seconds
- Practise five minutes of relaxation to create air shortage
- CP + 10 seconds
- Practise five minutes of relaxation to create air shortage
- Wait five minutes and measure your final CP. Your final CP should be twenty percent higher than at the start.

CP + 5 seconds. For example, if your CP is 10 seconds, then CP+5 seconds amounts to a breath hold of 15 seconds. Initially, it is better to do this when you are not distracted. Go to a quiet room. Turn off your mobile phone. Over time, you will be able to allow your breathing to relax and become quiet in any situation.

Another option for you is to listen to the attached CD, which is designed to instil relaxation and to guide you through reduced breathing. Listen to this CD before you go to bed. It is twenty minutes in length. While listening, ensure that you feel a tolerable air shortage for the entire twenty minutes.

Chief, how do you know if you are reducing your breathing?

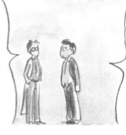

I feel relaxed and calm.

No, that is not correct.

You are reducing your breathing when you feel a tolerable need for air.

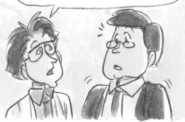

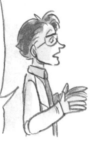

With each breath that you take, imagine that you are retaining CO2 inside your body. Breathe quietly to avoid exhaling all of that precious gas.

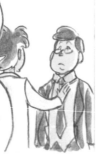

You can understand the importance of this gas by reading book two.

What body changes take place when you reduce your breathing?

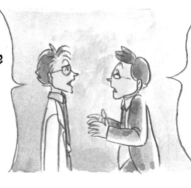

I cannot remember.

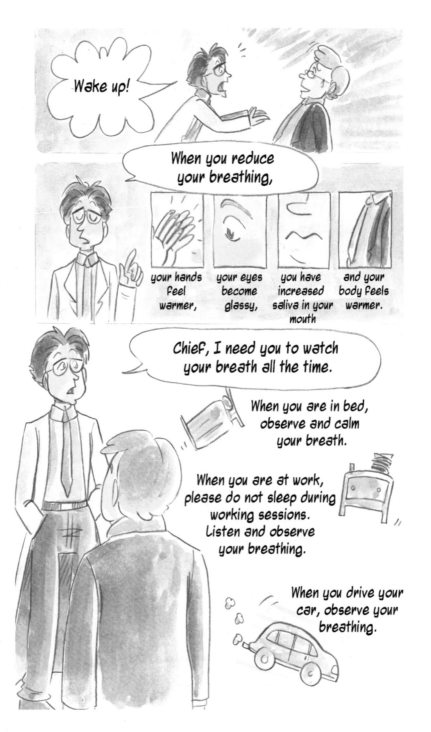

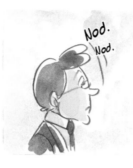

Nod.
Nod.

Throughout the day, ensure that your breathing is relaxed and calm.

Don't give in to heavy breaths, such as sighs or mouth gulps.

One sigh every few minutes is enough to maintain the habit of over breathing.

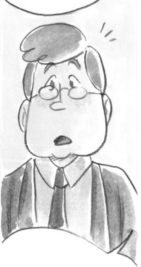

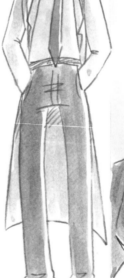

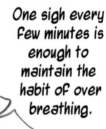

If you feel like you want to sigh,

swallow or hold your breath to avoid the large breath.

SUMMARY

- Try not to deliberately interfere with your breathing by tensing your muscles to breathe less

- Instead use mental commands and encouragement to reduce your breathing

- Incorporate reduced breathing through relaxation into your way of life

- Be aware of your breathing throughout the day

- Eliminate sighs and breaths through the mouth

REVERSING INSOMNIA

Buteyko: "Our lives are so busy and so frantic with tens of thousands of thoughts each day that the mind never gets a break. This madness increases our breathing and creates insomnia, but since everyone is caught up in it, few see it for what it truly is. So, it is good to devote twenty minutes to yourself every day."

By observing your breathing, relaxing your inner body, and allowing your breathing to reduce, the carbon dioxide level in your body can increase towards a normal level and brain cell excitability calms. In addition, the act of watching your breath is meditative and very helpful to calming the mind. You cannot think while you are relaxing your body and experiencing a shortage of air. Give yourself a holiday from your mind.

If you have never felt your inner body before, try the following exercise.

Place your hand in front of you. Now, close your eyes. Can you now feel your hand? Do you know whether your hand is there? Bring attention to your hand. Hold your attention there.

After twenty seconds or so, when you are sure that you can feel your hand, bring attention to your arm. With eyes closed, hold your attention on your arm.

After a period, bring your attention as far as your shoulder. Sense the energy vibrations as far as your shoulder. Feel the inner body. When you can comfortably hold your attention on your entire arm, gently move your attention across your chest.

Feel the inner chest. Sense the inner chest. Encourage this area to relax. You can help relax it further by physically tensing and relaxing your chest. Tense your chest and relax, tense and relax.

When you have a good feeling for your chest, bring attention to the area around your tummy. You can also help the area around your tummy to relax by physically tensing the tummy and relaxing. A very simple way to do this is to exhale and pinch your nose with fingers. Then try to gently breathe in and out while holding your nose to block airflow.

A stressed mind will always manifest in the tummy. Encourage this area to relax. Encourage this area to still. Encourage this area to be quiet.

When you have attention on the inner body, you will have stopped thinking. You cannot think and have attention on the inner body at the same time.

Humans are not simply made up of a head. Most people in the Western world are unaware of their body unless it feels pain. The only time that they bring attention to their body is when they are in pain. But your body is your connection with life. Realise this and disperse attention throughout your body.

As you go about your daily activities, try to identify the useless thoughts going about in your mind. Observe your thoughts. Be a passive observer. What are you thinking about? What purpose do the thoughts serve? Are they the same thoughts that you have been thinking for the past weeks, months, years? Are your thoughts beneficial? Do they help you or do they reflect the insane and repetitive nonsense that grips every Western human mind?

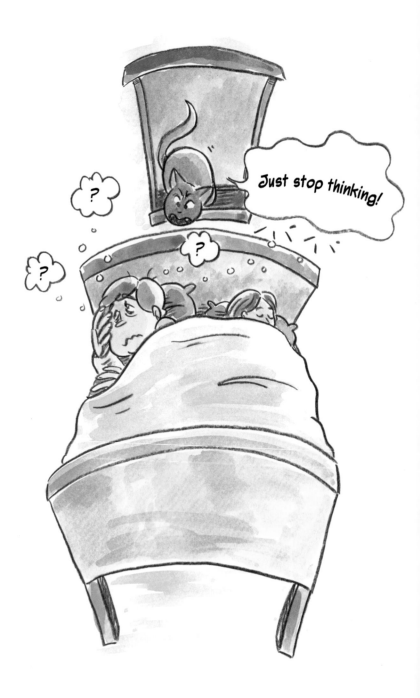

It is estimated that we have an average of sixty thousand thoughts each day. Furthermore, it is estimated that 90% of these thoughts are repetitive and useless.

An active mind with lots of thoughts is not so easy to switch off at night. If you have spent most of your waking hours investing in repetitive and useless thoughts, how can you switch that off when you go to bed? The more active your mind during the day, the more active it will be at night. This is why people often revert to alcohol and prescribed medications to help them sleep. But this does not work. Numbing the mind is no good, all it does it sweep the issue under the carpet.

The only way to stop useless thoughts is to address overbreathing and to make it a habit to still the mind.

BREATHING EXERCISE TO CALM THE MIND AND STOP PANIC ATTACK

Buteyko explained to Chief a very simple exercise to calm the mind or breath, called many small breath holds.

Sometimes, if there is so much agitation in the mind or the breathing drive is quite strong, holding our attention on the inner body or reducing our breathing might not be so easy. However, this exercise works very well as it calms everything.

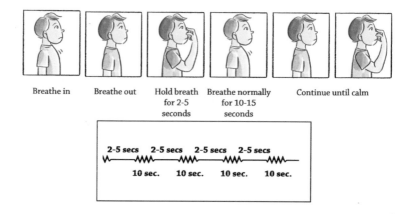

Breathe in   Breathe out   Hold breath   Breathe normally   Continue until calm
                             for 2-5   for 10-15
                             seconds   seconds

Do Many Small Breath Holds of two to five seconds each, as follows.

- Breathe in, breathe out, and hold your breath.
- Hold your breath for two to five seconds.
- After each breath hold, breathe normally for 10 to 15 seconds. Don't interfere with your breathing.
- Continue to do a small breath hold followed by gentle breathing for 10 to 15 seconds until your mind has calmed.

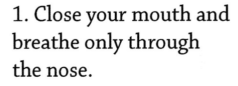

Remember, the Buteyko Method is about applying three principles:

1. Close your mouth and breathe only through the nose.

2. Adopt the correct posture.

3. Relax the inner body and create a tolerable need for air.

CORRECT BREATHING DURING PHYSICAL EXERCISE

Chief: "So Buteyko, does that mean that I don't have to do the exercise while sitting. Can you make the same progress while exercising?"

Buteyko: "Yes, you can. In fact, there are only two ways to increase carbon dioxide in the lungs. The first is by reducing the breathing volume and the second is by partaking in more physical exercise. Carbon dioxide is the end product from our metabolism, so the more we move our muscles the more carbon dioxide we generate.

Applying the three tenets to physical exercise will ensure maximum progress.

While exercising, **stand up straight** and imagine that a string of thread is gently lifting you up from the top of the back of your head. Breathe only through your nose and relax your chest and tummy."

As you walk, jog or run with your mouth closed, continue to **relax the inner body**. In particular, relax the area around your chest and tummy. Use mental commands to tell your body to relax. This is the exact same process as reducing your breathing while sitting.

The objective is to **create a need for air.** Ensure that you walk at a pace that lets you keep your mouth closed. To make progress, breathing should always be through the nose. Breathing must be controlled and the air shortage should not be so much that it causes you to open the mouth. If you need to open your mouth during physical exercise, you are pushing yourself too hard. Slow down instead and exercise at a level that is right for you.

Buteyko: It does not matter what sort of physical exercise you do. Ideally, you feel breathless, your breathing is controlled and through your nose, and you move enough to produce a sweat. Window shopping isn't much help.

You know that you are breathing correctly during physical exercise if your CP as measured half an hour after you complete your exercise is higher than it was before you began.

Another benefit of physical exercise is that it tires your body. You always sleep better when you are physically tired.

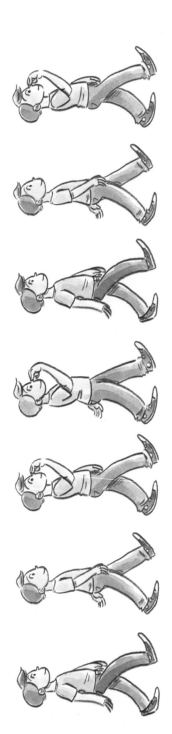

5-20 steps — 1/2 min. — 5-20 steps — 1/2 min. — 5-20 steps — 1/2 min.

The above is an excellent exercise for children and teenagers who may not grasp the concept of reduced breathing through relaxation. Further information on applying the Buteyko Method for children is available from www.ButeykoKids.com

74

Breath holds during physical exercise

This exercise is best suited for children, teenagers and adults in relative good health. If your CP is less than ten seconds or if you have any heart complaints, high blood pressure or moderate to severe sleep apnoea; it is advisable not to practise this exercise.

To do this exercise:

- Breathe in

- Breathe out

- Pinch your nose with your fingers

- While holding your breath, walk up to twenty paces

- When you release, let go and calm your breathing immediately

- Walk normally with your mouth closed for between half a minute and one minute to recover, and repeat again

- Repeat this medium breath hold every minute during a twenty-minute walk

YOU ARE ON AN AIR DIET

Chief met up with his secretary. This person was very much like Chief. Both were big people with rounded bellies, and who gorged themselves and were too lazy to do physical exercise.

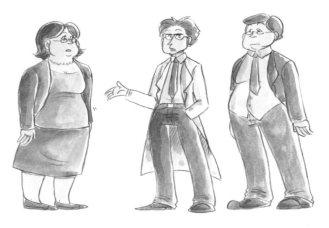

Chief: "I have someone for you to meet. His name is Buteyko and he has some advice with regard to eating."

As always, Buteyko was his usual direct self.

Buteyko: "Why are you overweight?"

Secretary: "I don't know. It is hereditary. I have always been overweight."

Buteyko: "Have you ever seen a fat person during a famine?"

Secretary: "No, that is a stupid question. How could one be fat during a famine?"

Buteyko: "That is correct. You are fat simply because you eat too much.

However, I am not going to waste your time by putting you on a food diet. That requires too much will power. Instead, I will put you on an air diet."

Chief and Secretary: "An air diet!!!"

Buteyko: "The ironic thing that most people fail to realise is that when you correct your breathing volume, your metabolic processes improve and the gastrointestinal tract receives more oxygen. Your need for food diminishes. Your appetite will change and normalise."

"Then you are not depriving yourself of food. You are not going on a crash or fad diet. In addition, with healthy breathing, your sleep is better, your energy levels are better, and you require less food. With less food, you will lose weight easily and effortlessly."

The best way to lose weight is to reduce your breathing to a normal level and listen to your body:

○ **Eat when you are hungry**

○ **Eat until you are satisfied**

○ **Finally, do not eat three hours before you go to bed**

Buteyko: "Look at this word: Breakfast."

"Divide the word: break fast. It means that our first meal in the morning is required, as we have been fasting from the day before. In other words, it is natural to wake up with an appetite."

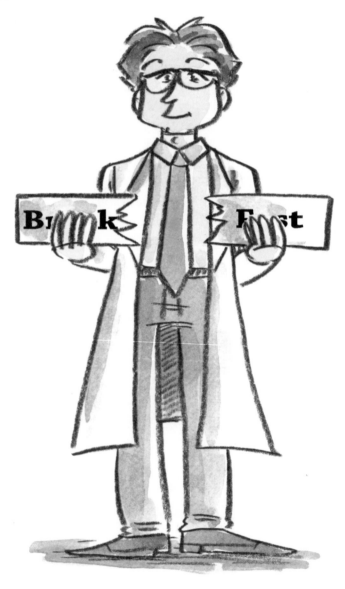

"However, if you gorge yourself before sleeping, you will not wake up hungry. You will still be digesting the food that you ate the night before. Eating and drinking alcohol late at night only creates insomnia."

"And here is another word that you are fond of: desserts."

"I would like you to spell it backwards."

Secretary: "Stressed. Wow."

Buteyko: "And that is how you are feeling. Too many desserts are contributing to your stress!"

Finally, avoid foods that produce symptoms such as nasal obstruction, increased mucus, and reflux. Typically, these foods are dairy, stimulants, and sugars. As your control pause increases, all three symptoms will greatly reduce in severity.

However, breathing is far more important than diet. Give your breathing 100 times more attention than your diet.

SLEEPING TIPS

B uteyko tells Chief that as his CP increases, his sleep will be deeper and his need for sleep will lessen. He quotes German philosopher Friedrich Nietzsche who once said that *"Sleeping is no mean art: for its sake one must stay awake all day."*

- In this vein, avoid taking naps during the day, as naps make you less tired at night and you will find getting to sleep difficult.

- Only sleep when absolutely necessary.

- Get up a half an hour earlier than you normally do.

You will not be more tired. Instead, you will be suitably tired so that when you do go to bed, you fall asleep easily.

Chief: "In addition, here are a few pointers for the bedroom. They are small points that can make a big difference in how you feel."

1. If your symptoms are severe, you need to interrupt your sleep every three hours. If you go to bed at 12 p.m., then set an alarm clock to wake yourself up at 3 a.m. When you wake up, check your breathing. If it is quiet then go back to sleep. If it is heavy, then it is very important that you sit up and do many small breath holds until your breathing becomes calm. When symptoms are severe, it is better to sleep upright in a chair instead of lying down. This might seem inconvenient, but needing a CPAP and falling asleep throughout the day is far more inconvenient.

2.   Your bedroom should be cool. A bedroom that is too warm and stuffy will make you breathe heavier. Ideally, leave the bedroom window slightly open even during winter. This will help keep your breathing calm.

3.   Do not eat for three hours before bed.

4.   With mild to moderate symptoms, sleep on your left-hand side or tummy.
      When you sleep on your tummy or left-hand side, your breathing volume is quieter. You will also experience far less sleep apnoea, snoring and heartburn, which is a contributory factor to insomnia.

5.   The worst position to sleep is on your back. Sleeping on your back causes the jaw to fall back in on the airway. This results in apnoea. Sleeping on your back also causes heavier breathing.

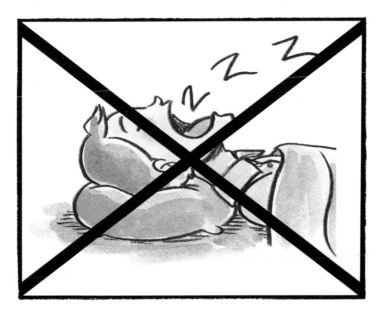

6. Do not watch the news or any other program involving negativity, stress, or violence before you go to bed. Instead, relax and reduce your breathing by listening to the CD that came with this book.

ARE YOU MOTIVATED TO MAKE THE CHANGE?

Buteyko had no doubts that both Chief and his secretary would make excellent progress. However, would they be motivated enough? Have they suffered enough to do something positive about their health? Or are they looking for a quick fix, like most of Western society?

His final reminder to motivate the two of them was as follows;

Buteyko: Your health condition is costing you time and, in your world, time is money. Your productivity is very poor. Your concentration is dreadful. Your mood is terrible. Your lifestyle is having terrible repercussions on your health. At the moment, you are working on half power.

Spend a little time to address your chronic overbreathing and I can assure you that it will be your best investment ever!

WHAT TO DO

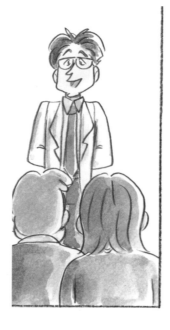

First and foremost, do what it takes to increase your control pause. I want you both to do the following.

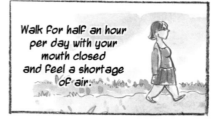

Listen to the accompanying CD once in the morning and once before going to bed at night. While listening, allow your body to relax, let your breathing reduce, and feel a tolerable shortage of air.

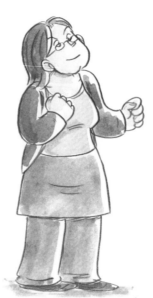

Walk for half an hour per day with your mouth closed and feel a shortage of air.

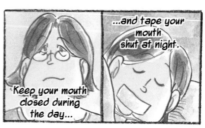

Keep your mouth closed during the day...

...and tape your mouth shut at night.

Spend ninety minutes each day reducing your breathing when sitting, by doing physical activity, or with many small breath holds. The following ideas may help.

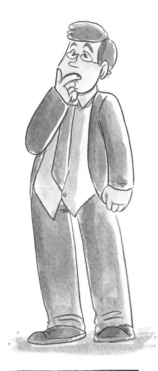

If you are stressed, do many small breath holds to calm your racing mind.

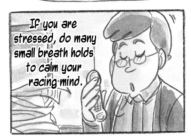

Keep bringing attention to your inner body and encourage your body and breathing to relax. Feel a tolerable need for air.

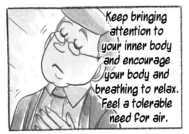

Adopt lifestyle changes such as eating when hungry, stopping when satisfied, doing physical exercise, and sleeping on your left-hand side or tummy in a cool bedroom.

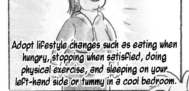

Finally, GOOD NIGHT.

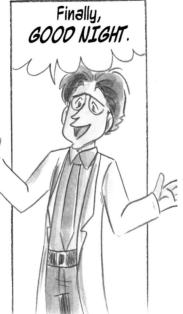

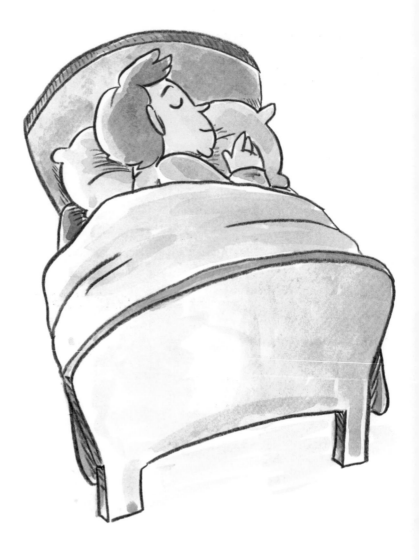

BOOK TWO

THE DISCOVERY

Excerpt from the book *Doctor Buteyko's Discovery* by Sergey Altukhov

It just seemed like an ordinary day. It was evening and Buteyko was on duty in a hospital, surrounded by a horde of noisy students who were also staying for the night shift. He was enthusiastically describing how his ideal doctor would diagnose illnesses.

"Just think," he stepped to one side to let past a nurse wheeling a trolley of medicines, "how do doctors mostly conduct an appointment with a patient? The patient has hardly come in before the doctor tells him to undress, turn around and breathe in." Buteyko acted it out to show what he meant. "We send urine, blood and faeces to be analysed." Buteyko turned his head away from the imaginary patient and handed an invisible sheet of instructions to one of the students. "No-one actually looks at the patient - no-one notices his eyes, the way he walks or his mood. But you can tell a lot from these things - sometimes almost everything."

Buteyko had only been working as a doctor for about a month, but he wasn't just sharing his own experience. He had absorbed the opinions of his mentor, Academician Dariev, who detested the overly formal and bureaucratic way doctors treated their patients.

"The patient is right in front of you. He hasn't said a word, but you can tell a lot about him. Here's a concrete example."

The Doctor turned to a well-built young man in grey striped pyjamas who was walking towards them with an awkward gait.

"Here's a typical asthmatic!" stated Buteyko categorically. "You can see that he swallows air like a fish."

The young man was indeed breathing with difficulty. The students glanced at each other in wonder. They liked this energetic teacher with his lack of vanity.

"I'm afraid you're wrong, Doctor," the patient croaked. "I don't have asthma, I've got malignant hypertension."

Buteyko saw the eyes of a dark-haired, pretty student cloud over with embarrassment and felt he was burning with shame. She had been gazing at him with such adoration just a few moments before.

"It can't be malignant hypertension!" exclaimed Buteyko as he followed the patient's slow progress along the corridor with his eyes. "That careful, restrained gait, shortness of breath, open mouth - they're typical signs of asthma. But he says he's got malignant hypertension. How could that be?"

The pretty student's face, flushed with discomfiture, and the hushed mutterings of the other students only spurred him on. Dr Buteyko's diagnoses were rarely wrong, let alone so short of the mark! Suddenly a thought flashed across his mind: what if the deep breathing that was typical of asthmatics and so pronounced in this hypertensive patient was not an external sign of the disease, but the reason for it? He felt dizzy with excitement. Saying he was urgently needed elsewhere, he sent the students away and hurried after the hypertensive patient.

A short conversation with the patient confirmed his nascent hypothesis. This 21- year-old patient was a weightlifter, which meant he inhaled and exhaled deeply as he squatted then lifted barbells. Buteyko remembered his own training. He too had lifted heavy weights and puffed like a steam engine. He had been forced to give up sport when he became ill, but he still breathed deeply.

Buteyko shut himself in the staffroom alone. The cramped room was dimly lit by a table lamp and outside it was dark. The window panes rattled slightly from the gusts of north wind. He had managed to leaf through about half of the patient's case notes when he felt a hypertensive crisis beginning. They usually came on in the evening or at night. He would feel the blood throbbing like a hammer in his temples, a sure sign of a sharp rise in blood pressure. The back of his head would feel as if it was on the point of splitting, his pounding heart would be seized with pain and his right kidney would ache. From habit, Buteyko put his hand in his pocket for the medicine that he always carried, then abruptly pulled it out again. What good was medicine if the underlying cause still existed? And that very evening, he had begun to suspect that deep breathing was the reason for his hypertension. So he needed to take the bull by the horns. 'Physician, heal thyself' echoed through his mind.

Buteyko laid the patient's case notes to one side. He took his hands from the desk, leaned against the chair's hard back, and began to breathe more shallowly.
No deep inhalations or strong exhalations, he told himself. Breathe as shallowly as possible. Just breathe a little.

He felt as if he was running out of oxygen. He wanted to open his mouth and swallow great gulps of air, but he restrained himself. A minute passed, then two, then three, and the miracle occurred. A true miracle. Buteyko's headache began to disappear and the pounding in his temples ceased. The pain in his heart subsided, leaving him feeling wonderfully relaxed. His aching right kidney felt as if it had been soothed with a hot compress.

"It worked!" Buteyko pushed up the left sleeve of his lab coat slightly. The yellow hands of his watch showed quarter to eleven. "It actually worked!"
Buteyko couldn't quite believe it. He deliberately took several deep breaths and his symptoms instantly began to return. He reduced the depth of his breathing, and the symptoms disappeared again.

He had been right! His hypothesis had been proven in a very concrete fashion.
He couldn't stay in the cramped staffroom a moment longer - he needed to confirm his findings using seriously ill patients! He was a scientist after all (albeit a young one) and knew that a successful experiment on himself was insufficient proof.

In Ward 14 on the third floor, Buteyko found an elderly patient who was blue from an asthma attack and looked as if he was about to lose consciousness.
Nurses were rushing around. They had already tried everything, including pure oxygen.

"Close your mouth and don't take long breaths," Buteyko ordered him in a deliberately peremptory tone.

"But I can't..." gasped the old man, trying to grab the rubber oxygen pipe from Dr Buteyko.

"Close your mouth!" urged Buteyko. "And press your hands to your chest." He crossed the old man's bony hands on his chest. "Stay as quiet as possible. Don't breathe deeply."

He gently pressed the patient's hands to his chest. In two minutes, the terrible bluish tone disappeared from the man's cheeks. He no longer grasped for the oxygen pipe, but instead gazed at Buteyko as if bewitched. The attack had clearly started to pass.

Until 3 am Buteyko visited as many wards as possible. Asthma attacks, angina, ischemia, and hypertensive emergencies all seemed to succumb to shallow breathing. Patients who had been rescued from terrible attacks stared at him in wonder as he left their bedsides.

At 3.10 am, Buteyko was again sitting at the desk in the staffroom. He hadn't put on the overhead light, but was using the old table light with its green shade.
The wind had started to die down and the window panes rattled less. The lampshade cast a shadow on the uneven surface of the wall opposite his table.

Buteyko had his elbows on the desk and his head cupped in his hands. The powerful technique that he had discovered that night had undeniably worked.
Encouraging a seriously ill patient to breathe more shallowly would bring him out of semi-consciousness and enable him to lead a full and healthy life.

Encouraging him to breathe more deeply would lead him directly to the Pearly Gates.

WHAT INCREASES BREATHING VOLUME?

B reathing increases as a result of our modern living style. Factors such as strong emotions, time urgency, tension, anger, stress, anxiety, overeating, processed foods, a belief that taking big breaths is good, lack of exercise, excessive talking, and high temperatures within the home all contribute to overbreathing.

HOW TO RECOGNISE HABITUAL OVERBREATHING

For most people, overbreathing is subtle. It is hidden, which is why it often goes undetected. The typical breathing characteristics of people attending my clinics include:
- Breathing through the mouth;
- Audible breathing during rest;
- Regular sighs;
- Regular sniffing;
- Irregular breathing;
- Holding the breath (apnoea);
- Taking large breaths prior to talking;
- Yawning with big breaths;
- Upper chest movement;
- Movement of shoulders while breathing;
- Lot of visible movement;
- Effortful breathing;
- Heavy breathing at night.

How many of these apply to you? Do you sigh? Do you breathe through your mouth? Do you wake up with a dry mouth in the morning? Does your breathing get faster or more chaotic when you are stressed?

IMPLICATIONS FROM OVERBREATHING

1)   Carbon dioxide, or CO_2, is a gas created as an end product from our metabolic process. The human lungs require 5% CO_2 or 40 mmHg. If we breathe too heavily, the partial pressure of CO_2 is exhaled or washed from our lungs. A loss of CO_2 from the lungs results in a reduction of CO_2 in the blood, tissues, and cells.

2)   Carbon dioxide relaxes the smooth muscles that surround the airways, arteries, and capillaries. With a normal breathing volume of 5 litres of air per minute, the partial pressure of carbon dioxide amounts to 40mmHg. Each 1 mmHg drop of arterial CO_2 reduces blood flow to the brain by 2%.[1] In other words, oxygenation of your brain significantly decreases when you breathe heavily. Lower carbon dioxide in the blood constricts the carotid artery, the main blood vessel going to the brain. The extent of constriction depends on a person's genetic predisposition but has been estimated by Gibbs (1992) to be as much as 50% for those with anxiety and panic attacks.[2] This finding is also supported by Ball & Shekhar (1997).[3]

3)   Balestrino and Somjen (1988)[4] and Huttunen et al. (1999)[5] demonstrated that CO_2 reduces cortical excitability. Cited in **Normal Breathing: the key to vital health**, "breathing too much makes the human brain abnormally excited due to reduced CO_2 concentrations. As a result, the brain gets literally out of control due to appearance of

spontaneous and asynchronous ('self-generated') thoughts." Balestrino and Somjen (1988) in their summary directly claimed that, "The brain, by regulating breathing, controls its own excitability."[6] In this vein, overbreathing is a significant and often overlooked factor in causing insomnia.

4)   During normal conditions, 75% of your oxygen intake is exhaled while breathing a healthy volume of four to six litres per minute. Even during intense exercise, it is estimated that 25% of our oxygen intake is exhaled. Breathing a larger volume than normal does not increase the amount of oxygen in your blood, as it is already 97–98% saturated. When one is overbreathing, carbon dioxide is removed from the body, causing oxygen to **"stick"** to haemoglobin within the red blood cells. This prevents its release into tissues and organs. This bond, discovered in 1904 by professor of physiology **Christian Bohr**, is known as the Bohr Effect.

5)   Heavy breathing volume during sleep causes turbulence and noise such as snoring. Drawing a large volume of air through a narrow space creates noise. Know that it is impossible to snore when the breathing is calm. Snoring is nothing more than very heavy breathing through the nose or mouth, or both.

6)   Heavy breathing causes the airway walls to collapse. It is not that the airways are too small, the problem is that breathing volume is too heavy. When the airway walls collapse, breathing muscles heave in an attempt to draw in more air. This only contributes to further holding of the breath constituting sleep apnoea.

BOHR EFFECT

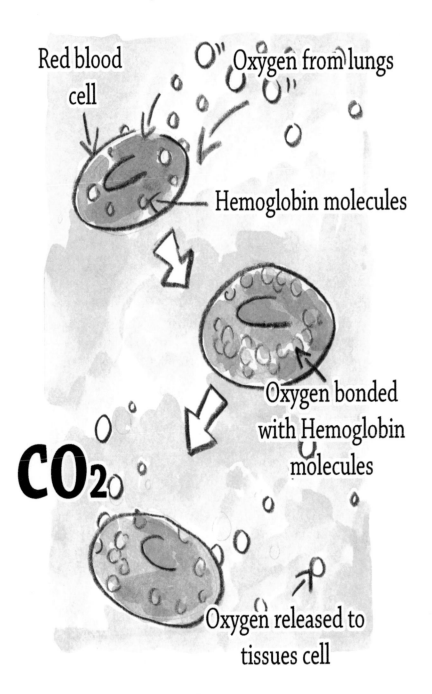

THE PREVALENCE OF SLEEP APNOEA

Sleep apnoea is increasing in prevalence, and this trend shows no signs of abating. In a paper published in the Chest Journal, Lawrence et al. wrote, "the demand for sleep medicine services has grown tremendously during the last decade and will likely continue."[1]

Studies have shown that a substantial proportion of the European and American populations have sleep apnoea. The American Lung Association estimates that about 12 million Americans suffer from obstructive sleep apnoea,[2] with the UK Sleep Apnoea Trust estimating 80,000 sufferers in the UK.[3] However, it is worth bearing in mind that these figures may not present an accurate picture, as some researchers claim that, so far, only one in ten patients with the syndrome are being diagnosed and treated.[4]

Forty offices and clinics in the U.S., Germany, and Spain participated in a study to obtain prevalence estimates for key symptoms and features that can indicate the presence of sleep apnoea in a broad range of primary care settings.[5] With a 78% return of 8,000 surveys seeking information on the prevalence of self reported chronic snoring, sleepiness, obesity, hypertension, and OSA risk calculation, one-third of participants were found to have a high pre-test probability for OSA, with a higher rate in the U.S. (35.8%) than in Europe (26.3%). Sleepiness affected 32.4% in the U.S. versus 11.8% in Europe.
Frequent snoring and breathing pauses were similar in both the U.S. and Europe (44%).[5] The paper concluded that "primary care physicians in the United States and Europe will encounter a high demand for services to confirm or

manage sleep apnoea, sleepiness, and obesity."[5]

The results from a 2005 poll to determine the prevalence of the symptoms and risk of sleep apnoea in the U.S. population, as published in Chest Journal, concluded that based on findings from 1,506 respondents, 57% were at risk from OSA.[6] The paper concluded that "as many as one in four American adults could benefit from evaluation for OSA. Considering the serious adverse health and quality-of-life consequences of OSA, efforts to expedite diagnosis and treatment are indicated."[6]

Kapsimalis et al. concluded from a study of 1,254 women in the U.S. that "twenty-five percent of the female population was found to be at high risk for OSA. (Obstructive sleep apnoea) "[7] Among women at risk, "habitual snoring (61%), observed apnoeas (7%), and daytime sleepiness (24%) were highly prevalent. Sleep onset insomnia (32%) or maintenance insomnia symptoms (19%) and restless legs syndrome (RLS) symptoms (33%) or body movements (60%) also were frequently reported. The risk increased with age, obesity, and menopause."[7]

Sleep apnoea is not isolated to developed countries. In a study to determine obstructive sleep apnoea among adults in Nigeria, Adewole et al. found that "overall, 19% of participants (22% of men and 16% of women) met the Berlin questionnaire criteria indicating a high risk of OSAS, (obstructive sleep apnoea syndrome)"[8] and concluded that "OSAS may be a more common medical problem than ever imagined among Nigerians."[8]

IMPLICATIONS OF SLEEP APNOEA (ADULTS)

- Excessive daytime sleepiness (falling asleep while eating, talking or driving)
- Waking up tired
- Bed partner is often worried about other health problems
- Patient may be unaware of own sleep disturbances
- Loud snoring
- Holding the breath during the night
- Loud snorts and gasps upon the resumption of breathing
- May cause marital problems
- Sometimes dry throat, dry mouth, and headache in morning
- Problems with memory and concentration
- Morning or night headaches affect approximately 50% of patients
- Heartburn or reflux
- Swelling of the legs
- Needing to urinate during the night
- Sweating during sleep
- Chest pain
- Temporary elevations in blood pressure
- Blood oxygen desaturation
- Arousal from sleep
- Sympathetic activation
- Can cause elevated blood pressure during the day, possibly leading to hypertension and heart disease

IMPLICATIONS SLEEP APNOEA (CHILDREN)

Children younger than five years of age

- Frequently waking up

- Snoring

- Sweating

- Mouth breathing

- Restlessness

Over five years of age

- Snoring

- Short attention span

- Poor academic performance

- Behavioural problems

- Bed wetting

- Not growing as quickly as they should be for their age

CPAP COMPLIANCE

The normal treatment for obstructive sleep apnoea is a CPAP (continuous positive airway pressure) machine. The patient wears a mask over the face and air is applied at a pressure that exceeds the airway opening pressure, thereby enabling the patient to breathe without cessation. In simple terms, it may be best understood as a small vacuum cleaner working in reverse, applying sufficient air pressure to force the airways open.

The CPAP can resolve apnoea in many patients, leading to improved sleep quality, decreased sleepiness, and lower blood pressure.[1,2,3,4]

The machine helps the patient as long as he or she continues to use it. On the downside, it does nothing to address the major contributory factor of sleep apnoea, namely chronic overbreathing. Wearing a mask during sleep can be claustrophobic, uncomfortable, cumbersome, and inconvenient, and getting tangled in the tube can be annoying. The air is very dry, which may cause rhinitis, a dripping nose, a blocked nose, and nasal irritation. Even when the mask is worn correctly, the feeling of the airflow is often described as putting ones head out of a car window while the car is moving at 30 miles per hour. Partners and patients often find the humming of the machine very distracting. The machine has to be cleaned on a regular basis, but few do this. Overall, while it is accepted as the gold standard of treatment, the CPAP machine has major short comings.

During one study of 300 patients referred to the London Chest Ventilatory support unit, it was found that 96% of patients complained of at least one side effect resulting from the therapy, while 45% complained of a side effect from the nasal mask.[5]

In a study of 80 patients, Verse et al. found that the most prevalent side effects were disturbance of the mask during the night (71.3%), dry mouth (47.5%), dry nose (46.3%), pressure marks from the mask (41.3%), crusts within the nasal cavity (38.8%), and hearing loss (26.3%). Mouth and nose dryness were considered the most irritating side effects.[6]

In another study of 41 patients with OSA, the paper noted that "the most frequently reported problems were a tender region on the bridge of the nose and discomfort associated with a dry nasal mucosa. Although CPAP treatment was initially accepted by most patients, adverse effects and other difficulties decreased patient compliance, with time, in many cases."[7]

A paper published in The Canadian Respiratory Journal observed that "compliance is a significant problem and has been incompletely assessed in long-term studies." After evaluating 80 patients to determine long-term compliance with CPAP, the authors concluded that "although many patients with OSA derive subjective benefit from, and adhere to treatment with CPAP, a significant proportion of those so diagnosed either do not initiate or eventually abandon therapy."[8]

The journal Sleep found that only 40% of the 162 newly diagnosed patients who required CPAP therapy accepted the treatment. The paper noted that compliance was higher in higher socioeconomic groups than the lower.[9]

Other researchers found that "failure to comply with treatment has been reported to be as high as 25 to 50%, with patients typically abandoning therapy during the first 2 to 4 weeks of treatment."[10]

According to Broström A et al., "Adherence to CPAP treatment is a multifaceted problem including patient, treatment, condition, social, and healthcare related factors. Knowledge about facilitators and barriers for adherence to CPAP treatment can be used in interventional strategies."[11]

WHEN CAN I STOP USING THE CPAP?

Thousands of individuals have eliminated their need for the CPAP machine after applying the Buteyko Method. How long this takes varies from individual to individual.

After a number of weeks of applying the Buteyko Method, improvement in your overall health and an increase in your CP, a suggested program for coming off the CPAP in conjunction with your doctor's advice is as follows.

- Go to bed without wearing your CPAP.
- Wear the tape to ensure that your mouth is closed during sleep.
- Set your alarm clock to wake you up two to three hours after falling asleep.
- Check your breathing when you are awoken by the alarm clock.
- If your breathing is heavy, then calm your breathing using the many small breath hold exercise.
- If your symptoms are no worse than if you had used the CPAP, try to fall asleep for the remainder of the night without the CPAP. If you wake up in the morning feeling no worse than your usual night's sleep with the CPAP?, then go to bed on subsequent nights without using the CPAP.
- If your symptoms are worse than usual, then use the CPAP for the remainder of the night.

During the following night, go to bed without the CPAP machine and repeat the guidelines above.

Please note: Do not make changes to the CPAP machine without consulting a medical doctor.

WHY HAS MY SNORING NOT REDUCED DURING THE WEEK?

The answer to this is whether your CP has improved. You won't feel an improvement unless your CP increases by more than 5 seconds. You need to place more attention on your breathing during the week.

- Are you breathing heavily?
- Is your mouth taped closed at night?
- Is your mouth closed during the day?
- Are you suppressing your sighs and yawns?
- Are you sleeping on your left hand side or tummy?
- Are you paying attention to reducing your breathing during the day?
- Are you breathing correctly during physical exercise?
- What is your lifestyle like?
- Are you talking all day?

Talking all day for a living is equal to breathing heavily all day. Hot temperatures, stress, processed foods, etc. all causes heavy breathing.

If you have a lot of factors causing you to breathe heavily, then you need to work harder on your breathing to compensate.

MOUTH BREATHING, SNORING AND SLEEP APNOEA IN ADULTS AND CHILDREN

Here, we examine the literature to determine whether sleeping with the mouth open is a causal factor for snoring and sleep apnoea.

"Open-mouth breathing during sleep is a risk factor for obstructive sleep apnoea (OSA) and is associated with increased disease severity and upper airway collapsibility." The study which involved 52 patients found that "the more elongated and narrow upper airway during open-mouth breathing may aggravate the collapsibility of the upper airway and, thus, negatively affect OSA severity."[1]

In another study, 385 patients with obstructive sleep apnoea were examined through a questionnaire. Results showed that upper airway symptoms were common, with 61% of patients reporting mouth dryness, 52% with nasal stuffiness, 51% with dryness of the nose, 30% with sneezing, 24% with mucus in the throat, and 17% with a runny nose.[2]

Ohki et al. performed a study to determine the relationship between oral breathing and nasal obstruction in patients with obstructive sleep apnoea. The study involved 30 normal subjects and 20 patients with snoring or sleep apnoea. Researchers found that chronic nasal obstruction and resultant mouth breathing may induce obstructive sleep apnoea.[3]

In a paper entitled, "How does open-mouth breathing

influence upper airway anatomy?"[4], Lee et al. tested the hypothesis that open-mouth breathing during sleep may increase the severity of obstructive sleep apnoea. After an analysis of 28 patients, researchers concluded that "open-mouth breathing is associated with reduction of the retropalatal and retroglossal areas, lengthening of the pharynx and shortening of the MP-H in the upper airway."[4]

After reviewing texts and articles on Medline, The Centre for research disorders in Cincinnati, Ohio concluded that obstructive sleep apnoea, sleep fragmentation, and disturbed sleep often result from nasal obstruction.[5] The authors of the paper observed that "since breathing through the nose appears to be the preferred route during sleep, nasal obstruction frequently leads to nocturnal mouth breathing, snoring, and ultimately to OSA."[5] The paper advised that allergic rhinitis and other upper respiratory disorders should be treated more aggressively.[5]

A Polish study noted that children with sleep respiratory disorders wake up tired, with blocked noses, were breathing through their mouth, tire easily, have concentration problems, are irritated, and demonstrate hyperactivity that may resemble ADHD symptoms. The paper further states that "long-term disease leads to exacerbation of all-systemic symptoms, results in cardiovascular complications, induces developmental inhibition and cognitive dysfunction, and is responsible for school/social failures and reduced life quality."[6]

In a paper entitled, "The nose and sleep disordered breathing: what we know and what we don't know," performed an analysis of medical literature on the subject.[7] The analysis confirmed that "SDB (sleep disordered breathing) can both result from and be worsened by nasal obstruction." It was stated that "nasal congestion typically results in a switch to oronasal breathing that compromises the airway." Furthermore, "oral (mouth) breathing in children may lead to the development of facial structural abnormalities associated with SDB." The paper concluded that the change to mouth breathing that occurs with chronic nasal obstruction is a common pathway for sleep-disordered breathing.[7]

Mouth breathing was also recognised to be a factor in a study to determine the prevalence and association of sleep disorders and school performance. Based on a total of 1,164 completed questionnaires on children aged between 7 and 13 years, it was found that the overall prevalence of snoring was 38.9% with 3.5% habitually snoring. "Allergic symptoms, daytime mouth breathing, shaking the child for apnoea, restless sleep and hyperactivity were significant and independent risk factors and sleep-related symptoms for habitual snoring."[9]

A study was conducted to determine the risk factors of habitual snoring and symptoms of sleep-disordered breathing. Based on a study of 1030 children aged from 12 to 17 years, it was found that "habitual snorers had significantly more night time symptoms including observed apnoeas, difficulty breathing, restless sleep and mouth breathing during sleep compared to occasional and non-snorers."[10]

And finally, data from 248 medical charts of mouth-breathing children were analysed to determine the prevalence of obstructive sleep disorders in such children. It was found that 58% of children were primary snorers and 42% had obstructive sleep apnoea. The paper concluded that, "primary snoring and OSA are frequent findings in mouth breathing children."[11]

There is no doubt that mouth breathing is a significant causal factor for snoring and sleep apnoea in both adults and children.

ALLERGIC RHINITIS, SLEEP BREATHING DISORDERS, ADHD AND REDUCED QUALITY OF LIFE

Allergic rhinitis is an extremely common health problem affecting up to 40 million in the United States and between 10–25% of the World's population[1] with the actual prevalence varying within and among countries.[2,3,4,5]

Typical symptoms of rhinitis include nasal congestion, runny and itchy nose, and sneezing. The eyes, ears, sinuses, and throat can also be involved.

The impact of rhinitis and how it negatively affects the quality and quantity of sleep is underrecognised and undertreated. "Nasal congestion, which is one of the most bothersome and prevalent symptoms of AR (allergic rhinitis), is thought to be the leading symptom responsible for rhinitis-related sleep problems."[1]

This section examines nasal congestion and its effect on sleep and ADHD. I have cited quite a number of studies to alert readers to the widespread recognition of this relationship.

Craig et al. notes that "nasal congestion is associated with sleep-disordered breathing and is thought to be a key cause of sleep impairment in rhinitis. The end result is decrease in quality of life and productivity and increased daytime sleepiness."[7]

Other researchers observe that "patients with chronic diseases, including chronic respiratory diseases, usually have considerably impaired sleep quality that may increase the frequency of exacerbations and severity of symptoms, lead to difficulty in patient management, and reduce quality of life (QOL)."[8]

In a paper entitled, "A practical approach to allergic rhinitis and sleep disturbance management,"[9] Davies et al. comments that "sleep quality can be significantly impacted by nasal congestion. This may lead to decreased learning ability, productivity at work or school, and a reduced quality of life."[9]

This is further summed up by Ferguson, who states that allergic rhinitis "can lead to impaired nocturnal sleep, and this impairment results in daytime fatigue and somnolence, reducing both learning and work efficiency and decreasing quality of life."[10]

Treatment of children with ADHD and problem behaviour is commonly done with medication or stimulants. An opportune question to ask is whether this is the correct approach given the potential benefits from addressing allergic rhinitis and improving the quality of sleep?

Researchers found that 28.1% of Singaporean children snored and 6% habitually snored.[11]
"Atopy such as asthma, rhinitis, and eczema was the strongest risk factor for habitual snoring in Singapore, and the effect was cumulative." The paper also noted that "children attending psychiatric services in Singapore may also have sleep disorders, the highest prevalence being in children with attention deficit hyperactivity disorder."[11]

In a paper entitled, "Pediatric allergic rhinitis: physical and mental complications,"[12] Blaiss noted that allergic rhinitis has a far more negative impact on the health of the child than just a simple sneeze. "There are numerous complications that can lead to significant problems both physically and mentally in the child who suffers with allergic rhinitis. Under physical complications, recurrent and/or chronic sinusitis, asthma, and snoring impact children with AR. Sleep disturbances, poor school performance, and hyperactivity are all mental complications seen in many children related to their nasal allergies."[12]

In a study by Gottlieb et al., parent questionnaires from 3019 children were analysed to assess the prevalence of sleep-disordered breathing symptoms in five-year-old children and their relation to sleepiness and problem behaviours. Sleep-disordered breathing was defined as frequent or loud snoring, trouble breathing or loud, noisy breathing during sleep, or witnessed sleep apnoea.[13] The study found "parent-reported hyperactivity (19%) and inattention (18%) were common, with aggressiveness (12%) and daytime sleepiness (10%) reported somewhat less often. SDB symptoms were present in 744 (25%) children."[13] Authors concluded that "children with sleep disordered breathing symptoms were significantly more likely to have parent-reported daytime sleepiness and problem behaviours, including hyperactivity, inattention, and aggressiveness."[13]

Brawley et al. analysed data from 30 children to determine the prevalence of allergic rhinitis in patients with physician diagnosed ADHD.[14] The paper concluded that "most children with ADHD displayed symptoms and skin prick test results consistent with allergic rhinitis. Nasal obstruction and other symptoms of allergic rhinitis could explain some of the cognitive patterns observed in ADHD, which might result from sleep disturbance known to occur with allergic rhinitis."[14]

Authors of the paper entitled, "Attention deficit hyperactivity disorder and sleep disorder," note that "there is a clear correlation between ADHD and sleep disorders"[15] and "by improving these children's sleep, the symptoms of ADHD are diminished and thus avoid the need to administer psychostimulants, which have undesirable side effects that produce a great deal of anxiety in the parents of these children."[15]

In a paper published in the journal Paediatrics, researchers concluded that "inattention and hyperactivity among general paediatric patients are associated with increased daytime sleepiness and---especially in young boys---snoring and other symptoms of SDB. If sleepiness and SDB do influence daytime behaviour, the current results suggest a major public health impact."[16] "Children undergoing evaluation for ADHD should be systematically assessed for sleep disturbances because treatment of sleep disorders is often associated with improved symptomatology and decreased need for stimulants."[17]

Bearing the documented evidence in mind, having a good night's sleep is imperative to the health of every child and adult. Treating rhinitis is an absolute must in this regard. "Health professionals and school personnel need to increase their awareness of the ramifications of this disease and actively work to prevent deterioration in both academic achievement and workplace productivity."[6]

ARE ASTHMATICS MORE SUSCEPTIBLE TO SLEEP APNOEA?

For ten years, children and adults with asthma and other respiratory disorders have attended my AsthmaCare courses in Ireland and abroad. One striking observation is the number of patients who attend for asthma but who also reported suffering from snoring, sleep apnoea, and chronic fatigue.

This is not surprising given the physiological effects from chronic hyperventilation that contribute to narrowing of the airways and sleepdisordered breathing.

Breathing volume is greater when asthma is severe, poorly controlled or unstable. This will have a knock-on effect by increasing the severity of snoring and sleep apnoea.

This section examines the relationship between asthma and sleep-disordered breathing, which includes snoring and sleep apnoea.

It is estimated that there are 300 million people worldwide with asthma, and its prevalence increases by 50% every decade.[1] The relationship between asthma, snoring, and sleep apnoea is significant, with one researcher claiming that "approximately 74% of asthmatics experience nocturnal symptoms of airflow obstruction secondary to reactive airways disease."[2]

From a study of 244 asthmatic patients, Teodorescu et al. found that "37% snored habitually and 40% demonstrated high OSA (obstructive sleep apnoea) risk." A high risk of

OSA was determined by asthma severity, reflux and use of an inhaled steroid medication. [3]

Julien et al. tested the hypothesis that the prevalence and severity of sleep apnoea is greater among patients with severe asthma compared with moderate asthma and controls without asthma. Comparisons were made between 26 patients with severe asthma, 26 patients with moderate asthma, and 26 patients without asthma of similar age and body mass index. The study found that 88% of patients in the severe asthma group, 58% of patients in the moderate asthma group, and 31% of patients in the controls without asthma group had more than 15 apnoeic events per hour. The paper concluded that "Obstructive sleep apnoea-hypopnea was significantly more prevalent among patients with severe compared with moderate asthma, and more prevalent for both asthma groups than controls without asthma."[4]

Researchers investigated whether asthma can promote obstructive sleep apnoea by examining the prevalence of OSA among patients with asthma that is difficult to control. The paper, published in The Journal of Asthma, concluded that the "study showed an unexpectedly high prevalence of OSA among patients with unstable asthma receiving long-term chronic or frequent burst of oral corticosteroid therapy."[5]

Similar findings were published in a paper entitled, "Association of Obstructive Sleep Apnoea Risk With Asthma Control in Adults," which found from a study of 472 asthmatic patients that poorly controlled asthma resulted in a threefold increase in the risk of obstructive sleep apnoea. The paper concluded "that there is a higher risk of OSA in patients with not well controlled asthma independent of known asthma aggravators."[6]

In a paper entitled, "Obstructive sleep apnoea syndrome and asthma: what are the links?" Alkhalil et al. noted that several studies confirm that asthmatics are more prone to developing obstructive sleep apnoea. The paper further noted that symptoms in common for asthma and OSA included nasal obstruction, a decrease in the pharyngeal cross sectional area, and an increase in upper airway collapsibility.[7]

DOES THE SLEEPING POSITION AFFECT SNORING AND SLEEP APNOEA?

Konstantin Buteyko discovered that the best position to sleep was on the left hand side or on the tummy. Ventilation is reduced while sleeping on the lefthand side given the position of the heart and on the tummy given the weight of the body restricting breathing.

Many studies show that sleeping on the back (supine position) is most contributory to snoring and sleep apnoea for both children and adults. Here, we examine available research.

Pereira et al. conducted research to determine the effect of body position on sleep apnoea in children younger than three years. Polysomnographies of 60 children were analysed for data on respiratory disturbance index, time spent in each position, number of apnoeic episodes in each position, oxygen saturation, and time spent in each stage of sleep. Researchers concluded that "there is an increase in the RDI (respiratory disturbance index) with increased time spent in supine sleep in very young children with obstructive sleep apnoea."[1]

A study of fifty children, 31 with habitual snoring and 19 with obstructive sleep apnoea, found that there were more apnoea hypopnea events when patients slept on their backs as opposed to on their sides.[2]

Davvat et al. assessed 430 children with obstructive sleep apnoea. The effect of different sleeping positions was examined in obstructive sleep apnoea, and in relation to obesity and tonsillar size. Children with OSAS were found to spend more time than controls sleeping on their backs, and that apnoea index was significantly greater in the supine position than in the side position.[3]

During a study of 574 patients with OSAS that was published in the medical journal Chest, researchers found that there were at least double the amount of apnoeas/hypopnoeas when patients slept on their back rather than their sides. The paper concluded that "body position during sleep has a profound effect on the frequency and severity of breathing abnormalities in OSA patients."[4]

During an assessment of 2077 OSA patients over a period of ten years, it was found that 53.8% had at least twice as many breathing abnormalities while sleeping in the supine (back) position compared with sleeping on their side. The paper concluded that "since avoiding the supine posture (back) during sleep may significantly improve the sleep quality and daytime alertness of many positional patients, it is imperative to carry out a high-quality study to evaluate if this is a real therapeutic alternative for many positional patients."[5]

A Japanese study of 72 patients and published in the journal Sleep found that most subjects in the snoring group decreased snoring both in time and intensity while sleeping on their side versus sleeping on their back.[6]

Another paper entitled "Association of body position with severity of apnoeic events in patients with severe nonpositional obstructive sleep apnoea" and published in the medical journal Chest evaluated the apnoeic events of 30 sleep apnoea patients when sleeping in either the supine

position (back) or the lateral position (side).
The researchers found that "even in patients with severe OSA who have a high number of apnoeic events in the supine and lateral posture, the apnoeic events occurring in the supine position are more severe than those occurring while sleeping in the lateral position. Thus, it is not only the number of apnoeic events that worsen in the supine sleep position but, probably no less important, the nature of the apnoeic events themselves."[7]

Szollosi et al. found that sleeping on the side reduces the severity of central sleep apnoea with cheyne-stokes respiration. The researchers found that "compared with supine position, lateral position reduced the apnoea-hypopnea index in all sleep stages" and that the "lateral position decreased desaturation independent of apnoea type."[8]

MOUTH BREATHING DURING CHILDHOOD INCREASES THE RISK OF LIFELONG OBSTRUCTIVE SLEEP APNOEA

It is inevitable that a child with a blocked nose will breathe through his mouth. Mouth breathing children often develop poor facial structures such as undeveloped chins, narrow faces and nostrils, crooked teeth, sunken cheeks and eyes, and larger noses.

When a growing child keeps his mouth closed, the tongue correctly rests in the roof of the mouth, creating a U-shaped top jaw. In other words, the shape of the top jaw is the tongue.

A mouth breathing child is unable to rest his tongue in the roof of the mouth. As a result, his tongue rests midway or on the floor of the mouth. The result is a narrow and undeveloped top jaw that is set back on the airways, creating smaller airways and an increased risk of developing lifelong sleep apnoea.

In the words of California-based dentist Dr. Raymond Silkman, "The most important orthodontic appliance that you all have and carry with you twenty four hours a day is your tongue. People who breathe through their nose normally have a tongue that postures up into the maxilla (the top jaw). When the tongue sits right up behind the front teeth, it is maintaining the shape of the maxilla (top jaw) every time you swallow. Every time the proper tongue swallow motion takes place, it spreads up against the maxilla (top jaw), activating it and contributing to that little cranial motion. Individuals who breathe through their mouths have a lower tongue posture and the maxilla does not receive the stimulation from the tongue that it should."[1]

Posnick et al. writes that, "a long-standing forced mouth breathing pattern with open mouth posture is known to impact on maxillo-mandibular (Jaw) growth and be a major contributing factor to developmental jaw deformities."[2]

This is further discussed by Ahn in a paper entitled, "Treatment of obstructive sleep apnoea in children." Ahn notes that, "the impairment of nasal breathing with increased nasal resistance has a well-documented negative impact on early childhood maxilla-mandibular development, making the upper airway smaller and might lead to adult OSA."[3]

In a study of children with a long history of habitual snoring and obstructive sleep apnoea, a neurological clinical examination showed that snoring started very early in childhood, at 22.7 months, while apnoea onset was 34.7 months. The authors of the study noted that, "23% of children showed a failure to thrive." Children with sleep apnoea showed different craniofacial changes with the development of a narrower vertical face and reduced upper airway space. The study concluded that, "these results suggest that oral (mouth) breathing, that is present in sleep apnoea patients, is responsible of different cranio-facial anomalies."[4]

Finally, a study of 26 children was conducted to detect the presence of early bone craniofacial modifications in young children with a long history of habitual snoring. The study found that upper airway obstruction during sleep is associated with mild but significant craniofacial modifications in children complaining of habitual snoring.[5]

TRADEMARK QUESTIONS

Does any group or individual own exclusive rights to the Buteyko Method?
The Buteyko Method is a system of principles and scientific conclusions that are impossible to protect by patents or other legal means. There are no patents granted in Europe or North America.

Who are Konstantin Buteyko's relative?
Vladimir Konstantin Buteyko, Konstantin Pavlovich Buteyko's eldest son from his first marriage, is a living relative of Buteyko. He now lives in Voronezh and is continuing what his father began. His wife, Marina Mikhailovna Buteyko, is the head physician-methodologist of the Buteyko Center in Voronezh. Vladimir and Marina have two children.

Who is the wife of the late Dr Konstantin Pavlovich Buteyko?
Susanna Nikolaevna Zviagina is Konstantin Pavlovich Buteyko's second wife. She was still alive and was his official wife at the time of Buteyko's death. She has never participated in the affairs of the Buteyko Method. Other people using the sirname "Buteyko" and claiming to be Konstantin Pavlovich Buteyko's wives are the result of name changes and not marriage.

As a qualified Buteyko educator or practitioner, do I need an annual license to teach the method?
No, once you have attended recognised Buteyko training, there is no requirement for an annual "license".

Is a Russian patent of the Buteyko Method applicable outside of Russia?
No. A Russian patent is only applicable in the jurisdiction of Russia. It has absolutely no validity in the United States, Canada or Europe.

Does any person or group have exclusive rights to teach the Buteyko Method?
No one group has special rights to teach or administer the Buteyko method. There are many Buteyko clinics in Russia, including the clinic run by the late Dr Buteyko's son, Dr Vladimir Buteyko, and his wife. Their website is at www.Buteyko.ru. Dr Vladimir Buteyko is keen to keep the method freely available and does not want any single group or individual to claim monopoly rights.

FAQ

Why does my coach always instruct me to breathe in through my nose and out through my mouth?
Many common myths become enshrined and entrenched in our culture, even though it may not be known why. It is thought that the main benefit to breathing in through the nose and out through the mouth is to rid the body of toxins accumulated in the lungs. However, if the mouth is kept closed in the first place, fewer toxins will enter the lungs. It is known that particles brought in through the mouth, which arrive in the alveoli, remain for 60–120 days before being removed. The disadvantage to breathing out through the mouth is that moisture is lost. Turbinates within the nose trap moisture to reduce dehydration. Mouth breathing, however, does not do this.

My friend is fit, yet his CP is only 15 seconds. Why?
Even though your friend is fit, he is chronically hyperventilating. It is very likely that his fitness would improve if he reversed his heavy breathing. I often address this question through the following analogy.

> *Person One – Swims underwater for a few strokes and is gasping for air.*
>
> *Person Two – Swims underwater for four or five times the length that the first person swam.*
>
> *Which person is the fitter of the two?*

Most people will say Person Two. You can then explain that this person has a high CP, whereas Person One has a low CP.

If it is relaxing to take a deep breath, then how is it considered bad?
Yes, if you tense a muscle and then relax it, it feels good. If you take a big breath, you are stretching your thoracic cavity and relaxing it. This contraction feels good. However, the big breath also reduces your carbon dioxide levels, increasing cortical excitability and muscle tension.

Do I need to reduce my breathing all day?
No, you do not need to do so all day, but try to reduce your breathing for a few minutes whenever you can. It is helpful for you to be aware of your breathing all day. On average, you may take 20,000–30,000 breaths per day. This will depend on your CP. Ask yourself how your breathing is, is it big, noisy, and irregular or is it calm, relaxed, and gentle? Whenever you think of your breathing, reduce it. Any time you feel that you are breathing too heavily, stop.

Can I deprive my body of oxygen by breathing too little?
Applying the Buteyko Method will not deprive your body of oxygen. On the contrary, it is more likely that you are depriving your body of oxygen because you are overbreathing. You are breathing heavily until your CP is 40 seconds, which means that you can reduce your breathing until you reach this level. After 40 seconds, there is no need to reduce your breathing.

If I fill the room with carbon dioxide, would this help?
This is debatable. For one thing, your body will only tolerate carbon dioxide to a level that your respiratory centre can realistically tolerate. If your carbon dioxide levels are higher, you will breathe more heavily to eliminate the excess. Some trials have shown beneficial aspects to the inhalation of increased carbon dioxide, while others have not.

I do yoga and my instructor teaches me to breathe heavily. Why is this?

In some instances, I have met people who claim that their health worsened as a result of breathing exercises during yoga. It seems that this depends on the instructor. If the instructor encourages heavy breathing, then that is not good for your health. If on the other hand, the instructor encourages reduced volume breathing by using breath holds, gentle breathing and correct posture, then this is a beneficial practice.

If I am doing physical exercise, I can only go slowly with my mouth closed?

Yes, but the quality of your exercise while retaining carbon dioxide is better. If your CP is less than 20 seconds, then it is very important to keep the mouth closed, as one hyperventilates easily upon the slightest exertion. When the CP is greater than 20 seconds, it is more likely that metabolic increases of carbon dioxide are greater than its loss. You can keep your mouth open for a short period when your CP is high. To determine whether you are exercising correctly, your CP one hour after you exercise should have increased by 25%.

I feel a constant need for air.

Yes, this is because you are breathing heavily and are trying to take a large volume of air through your nose. As your CP increases, your volume decreases and your shortage of air will disappear.

It is very difficult to set time aside to do exercises.

If this is the case, then try to do your exercises informally. If you drive, read, watch TV or are waiting for someone, then adopt correct posture and reduce your breathing. Try to get a walk in each day. If your job involves physical labour then reduce your breathing wherever you can.

If I change the number of breaths per minute, surely that will correct my breathing.

No, it won't. Many breathing exercises are aimed at reducing the number of breaths one takes per minute. For example, a person with a low CP could take 20 breaths per minute. Assuming that each breath represents 500 ml of air, then the volume per minute is 10 litres. If the rate was reduced to 10 breaths per minute, then each breath may increase in volume to 1 litre. In this instance, volume remains the same, i.e., 10 litres.

How do I know what breathing exercises are beneficial?

If breathing volume is reduced, then one feels a need for air. As a result, the CP should have increased following exercise. If the breathing exercise results in a higher CP, then it is a good exercise.

What is the right-hand rule of the Buteyko Method?

The right-hand rule does not require your attention. The left hand does.

1) Comfortable posture. This is achieved by sitting at the corner of a chair in the horse rider position. Sit up straight. Relax your shoulders with your arms down by your side.

2) Right of carriage. The chair must not be too hard (deepen breathing) or too soft (not good for posture).

3) Feet under chair. Both feet must be tucked underneath the chair and the height of the knees must be lower than the diaphragm. Sit up straight with your head facing forward, not raised and not lowered.

4) Closed mouth.

5) Eyes closed but looking upwards as if looking out a window from the top of the head. Please note that the head must not be raised upwards, only the pupils.

What is the rule of the left hand?

1) Gradual

2) Reduction

3) Of depth of breathing (breathing less)

4) Relaxation of the diaphragm. It is very important that the diaphragm is relaxed. The diaphragm is relaxed through tension. First, draw your stomach in and feel the tension. Then let it relax. It is necessary to switch from upper chest to tummy breathing. This will ensure a relaxed diaphragm, as it will be used instead of becoming tense and rigid. As you breathe in, the tummy gently moves out. As you breathe out, the tummy gently moves in. The tummy area should always be soft. When the tummy is soft, the breathing will be more relaxed. If the tummy gets hard, then stop reduced breathing for a while and then return to it.

5) To create a slight need for air (must feel a slight need for air of no more than your CP).
Do little incomplete breaths. Imagine that your chest is a glass. Instead of filling the glass full of air, fill it three-quarters full.

What is the DVBM?

DVBM stands for Deliberate Volitional Breathing Method and is the original name for the Buteyko Method. The name was changed to the Buteyko Method following a suggestion to Dr Buteyko from Buteyko practitioners Chris Drake and Sasha Stalmatski. The method was sometimes called "The Siberian Method of Self Suffocation" by Buteykos' patients.

THANKS

As always, this little book is the result of valuable inputs from many people.

A special thanks to Callista Bennis, Carol Baglia, Eugenia Malyshev, Jan Leuken, Tom Herron and Eoin Burns for their suggestions.

Thanks to Alex Spence for permission to use extracts from the book Doctor Buteyko's Discovery by Sergey Altukhov.

Thank you, Rebecca Burgess from RebeccaBurgess.co.uk for producing the beautiful illustrations which are found throughout.

As always, Aurora Pérez Machío delivered the perfect cover. If you ever need a book cover or other design, she comes highly recommended and can be found at www.apm-graphics.com

Thank you CPAP machine. May the thousands of snorers and sleep apnoeics find this little book before they become too disillusioned with you!

Greetings to Lauren and Sinead. May you both sleep silently with your mouths closed!

REFERENCES:

Book one
1)http://www.telegraph.co.uk/health/healthnews/6342113/Britains-loudest-snorer.html

Book two
Implications from overbreathing

1)   Cited in *Multidisiplinary approaches to breathing disorders* by Leon
        Chaitow, Dinah Bradley and Christopher Gilbert. 0443070539
2)   Gibbs DM 1992 *Hyperventilation induced cerebral ischemia in
        panic disorder and effects of nimodipine*. American journal of
        Psychiatry 149:1589-1591
3)   Ball, Shekhar A 1997 *Basilar artery response to hyperventilation in
        panic disorder*. American journal of psychiatry 154 (11): 1603-1604
4)   Balestrino M, Somjen GG, *Concentration of carbon dioxide,
        interstitial pH and synaptic transmission in hippocampal formation
        of the rat*, J Physiol 1988, 396: 247-266.
5)   Huttunen J, Tolvanen H, Heinonen E, Voipio J, Wikstrom H, Il
        moniemi RJ, Hari R, Kaila K, *Effects of voluntary hyperventilation
        on cortical sensory responses*. Electroencephalographic and
        magnetoencephalographic studies, Exp Brain Res
        1999, 125(3): 248-254.
6)   Artour Rakhimov Ph.D, *Normal Breathing- The key to vital health*

The prevalence of sleep apnoea
1.   Lawrence J. Epstein, MD, FCCP and Paul S.
        Valentine, *Starting a Sleep Center*. CHEST May 2010 vol. 137no. 5
        1217-1224
2.   http://www.lungusa.org/lung-disease/sleep-apnea (3rd March 2011)
3.   UK 80,000 http://www.sleep-apnoea-trust.org/ (March 2011)
4.   http://www.lunguk.org/media-and-campaigning/media-centre/lung-statsand-facts/sleepapnoea#_ednref7)
5.   Netzer NC, Hoegel JJ, Loube D, Netzer CM, Hay B, Alvarez-Sala R,
        Strohl KP;*Prevalence of symptoms and risk of sleep apnoea in
        primary care*. Chest. 2003 Oct;124(4):1406-14
6.   Hiestand DM, Britz P, Goldman M, Phillips B. *Prevalence of
        symptoms and risk of sleep apnoea in the US population: Results
        from the national sleep foundation sleep in America 2005 poll*.
        Chest. 2006 Sep;130(3):780-6.
7.   Kapsimalis F, Kryger M *Sleep breathing disorders in the U.S. female
        population*. J Womens Health (Larchmt). 2009 Aug;18(8):1211-9
8.   Adewole OO, Hakeem A, Fola A, Anteyi E, Ajuwon Z, Erhabor G.
        Obstructive sleep apnoea among adults in Nigeria. J Natl Med
        Assoc.2009 Jul;101(7):720-5.

CPAP compliance

1. Pepperell JC, Ramdassingh-Dow S, Crosthwaite N, et al. *Ambulatory blood pressure after therapeutic and subtherapeutic nasal continuous positive airway pressure for obstructive sleep apnoea: a randomised parallel trial.* Lancet. 2002;359:204-10.

2. Hack M, Davies RJ, Mullins R, et al. *Randomised prospective parallel trial of therapeutic versus subtherapeutic nasal continuous positive airway pressure on simulated steering performance in patients with obstructive sleep apnoea.* Thorax. 2000;55:224-31.

3. Norman D, Loredo JS, Nelesen RA, et al. *Effects of continuous positive airway pressure versus supplemental oxygen on 24-hour ambulatory blood pressure.* Hypertension. 2006;47:840-5.

4. Shivalkar B, Van de Heyning C, Kerremans M, et al. *Obstructive sleep apnoea syndrome: more insights on structural and functional cardiac alterations, and the effects of treatment with continuous positive airway pressure.* J Am Coll Cardiol. 2006;47:1433-9.

5. Kalan A, Kenyon GS, Seemungal TA, Wedzicha JA. *Adverse effects of nasal continuous positive airway pressure therapy in sleep apnoea syndrome.* J Laryngol Otol. 1999 Oct;113(10):888-92.

6. Verse T, Lehnhardt E, Pirsig W, Junge-Hülsing B, Kroker B. *[What are the side-effects of nocturnal continuous positive pressure ventilation (nCPAP) in patients with sleep apnoea for the head-neck region?].[Article in German]* Laryngorhinootologie. 1999 Sep;78(9):491-6.

7. Kuhl S, Hollandt JH, Siegert R. *[Therapy with nasal CPAP (continuous positive airway pressure) in patients with obstructive sleep apnoea syndrome (OSAS). II: Side-effects of nCPAP therapy. Effect on long-term acceptance]* Laryngorhinootologie 1997 Oct;76(10):608-13.

8. Wolkove N, Baltzan M, Kamel H, Dabrusin R, Palayew M. *Long-term compliance with continuous positive airway pressure in patients with obstructive sleep apnoea* Can Respir J. 2008 Oct;15(7):365-9.

9. Simon-Tuval T, Reuveni H, Greenberg-Dotan S, Oksenberg A, Tal A, Tarasiuk A. *Low socioeconomic status is a risk factor for CPAP acceptance among adult OSAS patients requiring treatment.* Sleep. 2009 Apr 1;32(4):545-52.

10. Zozula R, Rosen R *Compliance with continuous positive airway pressure therapy: assessing and improving treatment outcomes.* Curr Opin Pulm Med. 2001 Nov;7(6):391-8.

11. Broström A, Nilsen P, Johansson P, Ulander M, Strömberg A, Svanborg E, Fridlund B *Putative facilitators and barriers for adherence to CPAP treatment in patients with obstructive sleep apnoea syndrome: a qualitative content analysis.* Sleep Med. 2010 Feb;11(2):126-30. Epub 2009 Dec 9.

1) Kim EJ, Choi JH, Kim KW, Kim TH, Lee SH, Lee HM, Shin C, Lee KY, Lee SH. *The impacts of open-mouth breathing on upper air way space in obstructive sleep apnoea: 3-D MDCT analysis.* Eur Arch Otorhinolaryngol. 2010 Oct 19.

2) Kreivi HR, Virkkula P, Lehto J, Brander P. *Frequency of upper airway symptoms before and during continuous positive airway pres sure treatment in patients with obstructive sleep apnoea syndrome.* Respiration. 2010;80(6):488-94.

3) Ohki M, Usui N, Kanazawa H, Hara I, Kawano K.*Relationship between oral breathing and nasal obstruction in patients with obstructive sleep apnoea.* Acta Otolaryngol Suppl. 1996;523:228-30.

4) Lee SH, Choi JH, Shin C, Lee HM, Kwon SY, Lee SH. *How does openmouth breathing influence upper airway anatomy?* Laryngoscope. 2007 Jun;117(6):1102-6.

5) Scharf MB, Cohen AP *Diagnostic and treatment implications of nasal obstruction in snoring and obstructive sleep apnoea.* Ann Allergy Asthma Immunol. 1998 Oct;81(4):279-87; quiz 287-90.

6) Wasilewska J, Kaczmarski M *Obstructive sleep apnoea-hypopnea syndrome in children [Article in Polish]* Wiad Lek. 2010;63(3):201-12.

7) Rappai M, Collop N, Kemp S, deShazo R.*The nose and sleep-disordered breathing: what we know and what we do not know.* Chest. 2003 Dec;124(6):2309-23.

8) Izu SC, Itamoto CH, Pradella-Hallinan M, Pizarro GU, Tufik S, Pignatari S, Fujita RR. *Obstructive sleep apnoea syndrome (OSAS) in mouth breathing children. [Article in English, Portuguese]* Braz J Otorhinolaryngol. 2010 Oct;76(5):552-6.

9) Sahin U, Ozturk O, Ozturk M, Songur N, Bircan A, Akkaya A. *Habitual snoring in primary school children: prevalence and association with sleep-related disorders and school performance.* Med Princ Pract. 2009;18(6):458-65. Epub 2009 Sep 30.

10) Sogut A, Yilmaz O, Dinc G, Yuksel H, *Prevalence of habitual snoring and symptoms of sleep-disordered breathing in adolescents.* Int J Pediatr Otorhinolaryngol. 2009 Dec;73(12):1769-73. Epub 2009 Oct 20.

11) Izu SC, Itamoto CH, Pradella-Hallinan M, Pizarro GU, Tufik S, Pignatari S, Fujita RR. *Obstructive sleep apnoea syndrome (OSAS) in mouth breathing children.[Article in English, Portuguese]* Braz J Otorhinolaryngol. 2010 Oct;76(5):552-6.

Allergic rhinitis, sleep breathing disorders, ADHD and reduced qualit
life

1) Storms W, *Allergic rhinitis-induced nasal congestion: its imp* *on sleep quality.*Prim Care Respir J. 2008 Mar;17(1):7-18.

2) Sly RM. *Changing prevalence of allergic rhinitis and asthma.* A Allergy Asthma Immunol. Mar 1999;82(3):233-48; quiz 248-52.

3) Von Mutius E, Weiland SK, Fritzsch C, et al. *Increasing prevalence of hay fever and atopy among children in Leipzig, East Germany.* Lancet. 1998;351:862.

4) Romano-Zelekha O, Graif Y, Garty BZ, Livne I, Green MS, Shohat T. *Trends in the prevalence of asthma symptoms and allergic diseases in Israeli adolescents: results from a national survey 2003 and comparison with 1997.* J Asthma. Jun 2007;44(5):365-9.

5) Lima RG, Pastorino AC, Casagrande RR, et al. *Prevalence of asthma, rhinitis and eczema in 6 - 7 years old students from the western districts of Sao Paulo City, using the standardized questionnaire of the "International Study of Asthma and Allergies in Childhood"* (ISAAC)- phase IIIB. Clinics. 2007;62:225.

6) Borres MP. *Allergic rhinitis: more than just a stuffy nose.* Acta Paediatr. 2009 Jul;98(7):1088-92. Epub 2009 Apr 17.

7) Lunn M, Craig T. *Rhinitis and sleep.* Sleep Med Rev. 2011 Feb 10.

8) Muliol J, Maurer M, Bousquet J. *Sleep and allergic rhinitis.* J Investig Allergol Clin Immunol. 2008;18(6):415-9.

9) Davies MJ, Fisher LH, Chegini S, Craig TJ. *A practical approach to allergic rhinitis and sleep disturbance management.* Allergy Asthma Proc. 2006 May-Jun;27(3):224-30.

10) Ferguson BJ. *Influences of allergic rhinitis on sleep.* Otolaryngol Head Neck Surg. 2004 May;130(5):617-29.

11) Chng SY. *Sleep disorders in children: the Singapore perspective.* Ann Acad Med Singapore. 2008 Aug;37(8):706-9.

12) Blaiss MS. *Pediatric allergic rhinitis: physical and mental complications.* Rev Prat. 1996 Apr 15;46(8):975-9.

13) Gottlieb DJ, Vezina RM, Chase C, Lesko SM, Heeren TC, Weese- Mayer DE, Auerbach SH, Corwin MJ. *Symptoms of sleep-disordered breathing in 5-year-old children are associated with sleepiness and problem behaviors.* Pediatrics 2003 Oct;112(4):870-7

14) Brawley A, Silverman B, Kearney S, Guanzon D, Owens M, Bennett H, Schneider A. *Allergic rhinitis in children with attentiond eficit/ hyperactivity disorder.* Ann Allergy Asthma Immunol 2004 Jun;92(6):663-7.

15) Betancourt-Fursow de Jiménez YM, Jiménez-León JC, Jiménez-Betancourt CS. [*Attention deficit hyperactivity disorder and sleep disorders].[Article in Spanish]* Rev Neurol. 2006 Feb 13;42 Suppl 2:S37-51.

16) Chervin RD, Archbold KH, Dillon JE, Panahi P, Pituch KJ, Dahl RE, Guilleminault C. *Inattention, hyperactivity, and symptoms of sleepdisordered breathing.* Pediatrics. 2002 Mar;109(3):449-56.

17) Domínguez-Ortega L, de Vicente-Colomina A *[Attention deficithyperactivity disorder and sleep disorders].[Article in Spanish]* Med Clin (Barc). 2006 Apr 8;126(13):500-6.

Asthma and sleep apnoea

1. Sidney S. Braman, MD, FCCP *The Global burden of Asthma* CHEST July 2006 vol 130 no. n0.1suppl 4s-12s
2. Bonekat HW, Hardin KA, *Severe upper airway obstruction during sleep.* Clin Rev Allergy Immunol. 2003 Oct;25(2):191-210.
3. Teodorescu M, Consens FB, Bria WF, Coffey MJ, McMorris MS, Weatherwax KJ, Palmisano J, Senger CM, Ye Y, Kalbfleisch JD, Chervin RD. *Predictors of habitual snoring and obstructive sleep apnoea risk in patients with asthma.* Chest 2009 May;135(5):1125-32.
4. Julien JY, Martin JG, Ernst P, Olivenstein R, Hamid Q, Lemière C, Pepe C, Naor N, Olha A, Kimoff RJ. *Prevalence of obstructive sleep apnoeahypopnea in severe versus moderate asthma.* J Allergy Clin Immunol. 2009 Aug;124(2):371-6. Epub 2009 Jun 26.
5. , Tov N, Solomonov A, Rubin AH, Harlev D, Yigla M *Difficult-to control asthma and obstructive sleep apnoea.* J Asthma. 2003 Dec;40(8):865-71.
6. Teodorescu M, Polomis DA, Hall SV, Teodorescu MC, Gangnon RE, Peterson AG, Xie A, Sorkness CA, Jarjour NN. *Association of obstructive sleep apnoea risk with asthma control in adults.* Chest. 2010 Sep;138(3):543-50.
7. Alkhalil M, Schulman E, Getsy J. *Obstructive sleep apnoea syndrome and asthma: what are the links?* J Clin Sleep Med. 2009 Feb 15;5(1):71-8.

Does the sleeping position affect snoring and sleep apnoea?

1. Pereira KD, Roebuck JC, Howell L. *The effect of body position on sleep apnoea in children younger than 3 years.* Arch Otolaryngol Head Neck Surg. 2005 Nov;131(11):1014-6.
2. Kim HY, Dhong HJ, Lee JK, Chung SK, Jung SC. *Sleep quality and effects of position on sleep apnoea in East Asian children.* Auris Nasus Larynx. 2011 Apr;38(2):228-32.
3. Dayyat E, Maarafeya MM, Capdevila OS, Kheirandish-Gozal L, Montgomery-Downs HE, Gozal D. *Nocturnal body position in sleeping children with and without obstructive sleep apnoea.* Pediatr Pulmonol. 2007 Apr;42(4):374-9.
4. Oksenberg A, Silverberg DS, Arons E, Radwan H. *Positional vs nonpositional obstructive sleep apnoea patients: anthropomorphic, nocturnal polysomnographic, and multiple sleep latency test data.* Chest. 1997 Sep;112(3):629-39.
5. Oksenberg A, Arons E, Greenberg-Dotan S, Nasser K, Radwan H. *[The significance of body posture on breathing abnormalities during sleep: data analysis of 2077 obstructive sleep apnoea patients].*

[Article in Hebrew] Harefuah. 2009 May;148(5):304-9, 351, 350.
6. Nakano H, Ikeda T, Hayashi M, Ohshima E, Onizuka A. *Effects of body position on snoring in apnoeic and non apnoeic snorers.* Sleep. 2003 Mar 15;26(2):169-72.
7. Oksenberg A, Khamaysi I, Silverberg DS, Tarasiuk A. *Association of body position with severity of apnoeic events in patients with severe nonpositional obstructive sleep apnoea.* Chest. 2000 Oct;118(4):1018-24.
8. Szollosi I, Roebuck T, Thompson B, Naughton MT. . *Lateral sleeping position reduces severity of central sleep apnoea / Cheyne-Stokes respiration.* Sleep. 2006 Aug 1;29(8):1045-51

YKO BOOKS, DVDS AND NE SELF HELP COURSES

sthma Free naturally by Patrick McKeown

Close Your Mouth by Patrick McKeown

Anxiety free: stop worrying and quieten your mind by Patrick McKeown

Doctor Buteyko's Discovery by Sergey Altukhov

Buteyko meets Dr Mew by Patrick McKeown

ABC to be asthma free by Patrick McKeown

DVD SETS

- ButeykoDVD.com set by Patrick McKeown

- ButeykoChildren.com DVD set by Patrick McKeown

ONLINE SELF HELP COURSES

- www.ButeykoDVD.com by Patrick McKeown

- www.AsthmaCare.us by Eugenia Malyshev

- www.CorrectBreathing.com by Carol Baglia